PREVENTION IS DIFFICULT – BUT POSSIBLE

ALLEN J. OREHEK, MD

ISBN-10: 1475017529
EAN-13: 9781475017526
Library of Congress Control Number: 2011945121
CreateSpace, North Charleston, SC

Enjoy.

CONTENTS

INTRODUCTION

"The cure is possible—*prevention is difficult*."
—Allen J. Orehek, MD

A note from the author: If some of what I say in this book surprises you, I will consider it successful. I not only present important and sometimes unpopular ideas but also present them with candor and—I hope—humor. I don't wish to offend anyone, but it's important to me that you see your author as he sees himself: a human being, with human experiences and a human outlook. With any luck you will simply see me as someone who gives you important information at a time of your need. So that we are clear, do not look to me to be "a good guy." I am here for you, and this is all about you. I have put thousands of hours of work and research into this project so that you do not have to. Most of the subject matter is controversial, and at times both sides of an issue can be correct. But I care deeply about this topic, and I don't wish to hide that fact. The most difficult part of writing a book is trying to know who is reading it. This book should go to press in seven billion different ways because everyone is unique. Your background and history will make your interpretation of what I have written slightly different from the next person's. When I have facts to back up my details, I reference them, and when I am sharing an opinion, well, I am opinionated. Enjoy.

About the title: While adjusting the title of the book, the word *cure* seemed to take on so many different lights that I was concerned that some people would misunderstand a subtitle of "The Cure for Alzheimer's and Dementia Is Possible." That was not my intention. If one considers the cure to be the elimination of a disease or condition with medical treatment or a means of improving a condition, then the cure for Alzheimer's and dementia is possible. All hope is not lost for those who already have the disorder, as mitigation of disease progression is at your doorstep. Cure, if considered as the act of preserving a product, allows an unintended additional relationship, as preservation of your brain is the main topic of some chapters. An untenanted lifestyle without any thoughts of prevention of disease will not lead to your cure.

Background: Most people can prevent Alzheimer's disease and dementia, heart- and stroke-related incidents, and cancers from spreading by asking their health care team to conduct tests that will show any proclivity to these events—even when they are currently not having symptoms. Health care teams are often unwilling to recommend these tests because they are subject to the standard operating procedures of health insurance companies. People could be unwilling to take these tests because they may have to pay for them out of pocket. Many tests, however, provide patients with valuable information about the state of their arteries, their organs, and their brains; patients and doctors can use this information to create a disease-prevention plan that can help them avoid disease states later in their lives. This is a new philosophy and way of thinking in medicine. A totally innovative approach to diagnosis and management of diseases awaits you inside this book. What you are about to read will be controversial, as links that are only partially proven can be considered speculative. Should any aspect of this information provide you an advantage in your unique life, then I consider the whole work a success. I am a doctor, but I am not your doctor. Most of the information I will provide is from a physician of medicine and not as a provider of health care. Only after many years or decades of research will the concepts in this book be tested to a point to be considered theory.

MEDICAL PREVENTION DEFINED: A new area of medicine that combines different concepts into a philosophy of medical care. It applies the science of medicine to the motivated and unique individual. Working at the level of the individual to detail prevention of disease states, Medical Prevention does not apply general guidelines that cover large populations. The concepts deal with medical care—not health care. It is sometimes controversial, as some links to prevention have only superficial evidence and the specific subject has not been completely evaluated or studied in medical science—that will take years.

SCIENTIFIC AND DEVELOPED APPROACH: This book is a scientific and developed approach for preventing diseases and cancers. At the top of my list of preventable diseases is Alzheimer's. Using the advice outlined in this book, a motivated individual will find new ways to prevent dementia. The philosophy of unique care proffered in this book will also help prevent stroke, heart disease, and cancers. Many of these diseases and cancers are found in the general population and are allowed to run their clinical course, causing pain and suffering. Allowing these diseases to take hold and flourish is incredibly expensive for patients and governments around the world. The cost of stroke and cardiovascular disease for the United States alone was estimated at $503.2 billion in 2010.[1] When one adds in the cost of the other disease states that are preventable, the total is in the trillions. Most dementia, for example, is absolutely preventable and treatable.

This is where this work will shine for you—a new understanding that dementia is preventable. Appreciate that point again: *your dementia is preventable* if you follow my advice.

THIS BOOK WILL SAVE YOUR LIFE: Who would not want to know everything they could do to save their own lives? I am not boasting here—I'll provide you with the supporting science and data. I will provide tools for your success. Then you can decide for yourself. You have to consider what you can do before a disease takes you, compared to what you have to do after the disease claims you. Often one wants to go back in time and do that short or easy testing that would have prevented the disaster of pain and suffering that one is now facing.

Yes, this book can save your life. You can also apply this process to your loved ones to prevent their pain and suffering from preventable diseases. There are almost seven billion people in the world[2], and only a small fraction of them are doing anything at all to prevent the diseases that will end their lives. Although you can add up the direct financial cost of illness and death, you simply can't measure the cost in pain and suffering to the individual and all those involved.

LIFE EXPECTANCY: At age seventy-five, your average life expectancy is about eleven years.[3] If you are a woman, you will average twelve and half more years of life, and as a man, about ten and half more years. With that much time left, you had better take good care of yourself! Even at age eighty-five, the average life expectancy is six and half years—so why would you allow preventable diseases from ruining your remaining time? You can add another seven years to those numbers if you remove major cardiovascular disease.[4] Your remaining time can be wonderfully productive and active. I have many patients in their eighties who lead satisfying and loving lives. Often they are still side by side and hand in hand with the one they have loved for many years. You also, if you work at it, can live fully every day you have on earth.

LIVE BETTER AND LONGER: Because you are reading this book, you will live better and longer. That is not a boast but a fact. I hope that when you are ninety-four years old, "chillin'" in the backyard with some lemonade, you will gratefully look back upon your life and realize how you were able to avoid so many preventable diseases.

DIE FROM OLD AGE: I have had patients die from old age. No cancer or no significant disease state overcame them. They just died. They began the day doing their regular thing. Some of them seemed as though they were waiting for something to happen before they passed. A special occasion or a visit from a unique person seemed to be "the end of the road," and they just passed on.

PROPER MAINTENANCE: I would like you to recall the last time that you purchased an item that required some aspect of maintenance to keep it operating properly. Usually, a simple procedure at a set interval keeps the item running and oper- ating perfectly. Every household appliance, every computer, and every tool comes with some instructions. Did you not ever wonder where the manual for your own body is? Did you lose that someplace? You do not have a sticker on your body re- minding you how to take care of it, I am sure. When one learns how to operate and maintain a piece of equipment properly, it runs better and lasts much longer than something left to its own process. Your body is the same.

In fact, the ideal way to conceive of your body is as a ma- chine. Your joints function with amazing physics, the connection of ligaments to bone creating fantastic leverage. Your muscles increase in bulk and size as a response to stress, strain, and train- ing. Your bones act like the support beams in the structure you are living within, providing strength and stability. When you push them too much, they break. I would be so excited to explain all of the workings of your internal organs, how they operate in response to chemical and electrical signals from inside the body—but you get the idea.

The honest downside of all of this is that many of us do not take good care of our bodies, and some people are even downright destructive. They may come to a crossroad in life and decide that it is time to do some maintenance, yet when they go for medical care, they get only a very rough draft of what they should be doing. You deserve better!

MONEY AND FAME: Money and fame do not guarantee good health, and even the most expensive and advanced treatments often can't stop a disease once it has started. Money and fame do not always get you good medical care. A look at the health of many recent world leaders—perhaps some of the most famous people in history—makes the point quite clearly. Ronald Reagan's colon cancer was diagnosed in 1985, and he died in 2004 after a ten-year struggle with Alzheimer's disease. John McCain's malignant melanoma was diagnosed in 1993 and again in 2000. Corazon Aquino, the first female president of the Philippines, received a diagnosis of colon cancer in 2008 and died after it spread to other organs. Charlton Heston publically explained he had "symptoms consistent with Alzheimer's disease" in 2002 and by 2005 had difficulty getting out of bed.[5]

Entertainers and athletes also fall into the same trap. Farrah Fawcett died at age sixty-two from anal cancer. Lance Armstrong received a diagnosis of advanced testicular cancer in 1996 at age twenty-five. Patrick Swayze died at age fifty-seven from pancreatic cancer. Sharon Osborne received a diagnosis of colon cancer at age fifty. Rod Stewart was age forty-five when he received a diagnosis of thyroid cancer. John Candy died at age forty-three of a heart attack. Gilda Radner died from ovarian cancer.[6] John Ritter died in 2003 from a ruptured ascending aneurysm. Mickey Mantle died from liver cancer. "Mama" Cass Elliot, at age thirty-two, "passed away after suffering a heart attack while sleeping."[7] Bob Marley died at age thirty-six from malignant melanoma. Daniel Paul Federici died at age fifty-eight from melanoma. Steve Jobs died from pancreatic cancer when his worth topped $6 billion.[8] Neither wealth nor notoriety prevents disease.

CURE IS COMPLICATED: Because the cure is complicated, I go into detail in almost every aspect. If you have a background in medicine or science, you may want further information. I would love to sit and have some coffee with you and show you that all of my facts are tight, my conclusions are backed by proof, and my reasoning is sound. The least expensive test is the one that makes the diagnosis. **Prevention is difficult**; the cure is complicated.

TOBACCO: If you use tobacco and don't plan to quit, then stop reading this book. This book is not likely to do you any good at this time in your life. The cure is possible, but not against the tidal wave of tobacco use.[9] [10] [11] Many people quit after a stroke, heart attack, or development of a cancer, but it's too late already for prevention. I do tell my patients, "As your physician I must advise you to quit tobacco." Your body is amazing and dynamic, and there is a chance that your immune system will detect any of the cancer cells you are creating. Perhaps you will not get a cancer. But if you could stop smoking, it would be the single best thing in your life to prevent a variety of diseases and cancers. Often patients have found some help when they started to think of their tobacco use as a "per puff" and no longer as a number of cigarettes or packs per day.

PSYCHOLOGICAL ABANDONMENT: When you go to the doctor, there is a good chance that you will be getting the "fast-food" style of medical care. This type of medical care mixes all of the people who seek preventive care with the ones who have no desire or plan for any type of prevention. If you take your car to the shop because you think the brakes are not working properly—they make a sound, feel soft, or 'don't apply fast enough—you expect that they will be repaired. And if the guy at the counter tells you to wait a while and bring the car back when the brakes fail altogether you would be, like, "WTF?" and really wonder what just happened. You might stand there for a second wondering if the guy is kidding or whether you have to now find another shop. When you go to your doctor and she pats you on the back, telling you that you "look good" and "you are doing fine for someone your age," when what she means is that she doesn't want to know the problems you have under the hood.

When we wait for chest pain, it is too late. When we wait for changes in the memory, it is too late. When we wait for a lump, it is often too late. When we wait for that mole to change, often it is too late. You are more than welcome to continue with the good old pat on the back and some reassurance that you are doing "great for your age," but I maintain that you simply have not looked at what is going on. How does a doctor know you are doing great when without a specific test he would not be able to detect a nodule on your thyroid that could be cancerous?[12] I'm sure he told you it is close to impossible for him to find it while doing an examination. It is not likely that he will offer you an ultrasound of your thyroid. Even if you ask about one, you will get a reference to some junk science that says, "Don't look and don't find anything."[13] I am sure that any physicians reading this book are mumbling, "Why is this guy looking for these diseases? Why bother? Why put people through any tests?" Well, I chuckle here a bit. What is so hard about doing an ultrasound? All it asks of the patient is skipping breakfast and driving to an image center.

Few people would be up to the task of discovering what their bodies have going on inside. I asked a new patient once when we first met, "Are you ready?"

She replied, "Ready for what?"

"Ready to find out what can go wrong before it goes wrong."

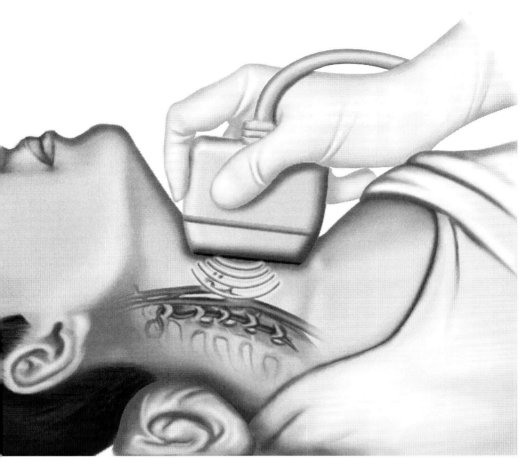

I am sure if you could to talk to people dying from met-astatic cancer pain, they would tell you they wished they had put in the time at some earlier point to avoid being in that horrible condition. Sometimes disease is unavoid-able. Yes. So at times these diseases come and take their natural course despite your trying to avoid it. But you can do much better at preventing than you have been doing. When you're done reading this book, or perhaps even be-fore you're done, you will discover part of the who and what that makes up you. You will want to get properly evaluated for Medical Prevention. Perhaps it is just that nagging fear of pancreatic cancer—but don't do it out of fear. Do it to take care of your body. Before you finish this book, you will be thinking about a plan to complete what needs to be done for preventing! Prevention is difficult only in the aspect that you have a lot of work to do. The concept and the wisdom of it are relatively simple. The prevention of your diseases should be as natural as having an understanding of your organs. Knowing what organs make up your body requires about a high school education. Do you know what organs make up your body? Do you know what disease process is killing the people around you? Do not fret as much with what is new and exciting; rather, stick to the basics of your organs. Yes, there are exciting genetic evaluations and detailed DNA testing. Before you go there, be sure to get an idea of the contour of your organs. Is there a solid mass inside it? No one will notice until it is pushing on something, so best for you to find it when it has not yet spread.[14] All cancer starts as one messed-up cell. The more it duplicates, the larger the mass, and once it invades the lymph system or bloodstream, you could be in deep trouble. You may not have much luck in detecting the first messed-up cell, but as a group of them forms a mass, you might be able to notice this before it spreads.

A country truly concerned with improving the wellness of its population will decide to integrate aspects of this book into its current health system. I doubt that the United States will integrate much of the needed aspects of this approach because far too much money is being made from the treatment of these diseases than could ever be made in their prevention.[15] Capitalism, as one of the foundations of the United States, will always encourage decisions based on someone's ability to make money and not on what is proper, right, thoughtful, or humane.

This book takes you through a number of the major diseases and what can be done to truly initiate widespread eradication and prevention of these disease processes. This book faces a significant amount of resistance because there are a large number of companies, organizations, academies, study groups, and people who make money from these disease states. One could agree that it is unfortunate that where money may represent a potential power, money in the hands of such corporations can easily squash the truth and put a turn on this book. When that occurs, the common person will never do much better than get a cancer, suffer a stroke, or develop a disease that she could have prevented. We should be able to enjoy our lives up to the day when we are sitting in our backyards, drinking lemonade, and pass away from old age, simply old age. I will not be able to fix, or will I even try to fix, the fact that many professionals know what needs to be done to prevent your mother's first stroke, but they will not tell you. You will not go to your doctor's office and find out what should be done to prevent her pain that is waiting. (This is your pain also because you will be the one taking care of her!) I know you love your mother, and I want you to find out how close she is to her first stroke. This is an easy thing to do—quite simple, actually. You will prevent it! I see billboards and advertisements that brag about how a facility treats and rehabs strokes ("11,000 strokes treated"). These facilities are bragging; they are happy these people have strokes because it keeps them in business. You should see *my* advertisement! A monkey can make the diagnosis *after* a stroke or ministroke. You don't need a doctor once this damage is done. It is over. The horse has left the barn! I hope the patient can make a good recovery, but it would have been easier to prevent this.

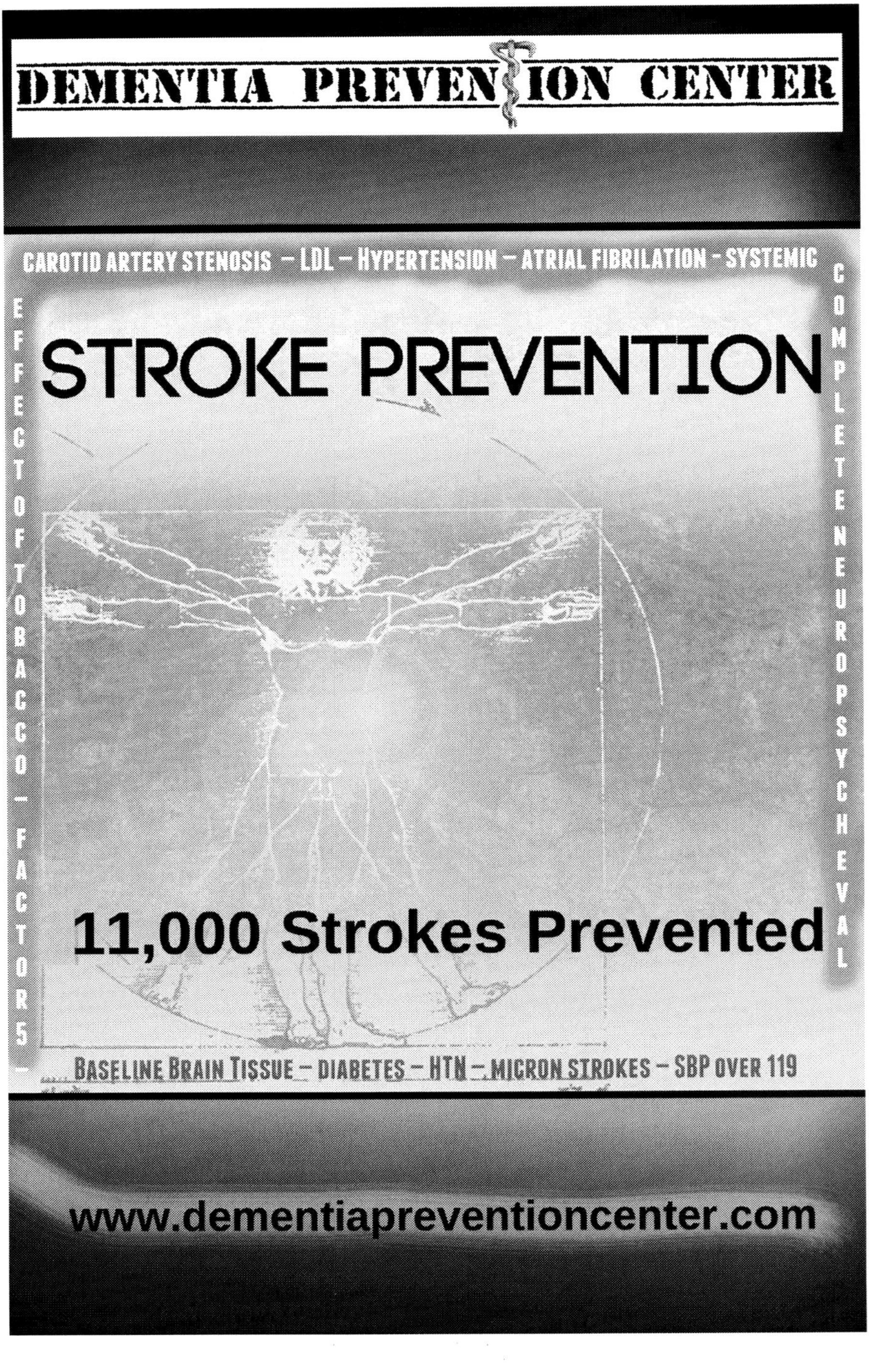
DEMENTIA PREVENTION CENTER
CAROTID ARTERY STENOSIS – LDL – HYPERTENSION – ATRIAL FIBRILATION - SYSTEMIC
EFFECT OF TOBACCO – FACTORS –
COMPLETE NEUROPSYCH EVAL
STROKE PREVENTION
11,000 Strokes Prevented
BASELINE BRAIN TISSUE – DIABETES – HTN – MICRON STROKES – SBP OVER 119
www.dementiapreventioncenter.com

If you are from another country or culture and you are reading this book, then you may or may not understand how things in the United States differ from things in your country. There are too many variables for me to be able to even tackle the aspect of your health care system and how it applies to the care that you get. However, as you read this book, you will be able to understand some of what happens in the United States. At times you may feel that it is better, and other times you may be happy with what you have in your home country.

The cure is complicated, but it starts with prevention.

When a test is completed, whether the results are good or bad often depends on the test. A test that diagnoses ovarian cancer that has not yet spread or a test that finds critical cardiac disease without symptoms is considered a good test. When one discovers that one has carotid artery stenosis of 10 percent and can start treatment before a *micron stroke*[16] occurs, this, again, is a good thing. If a test is completed and found to be normal, then you need to check back in with that organ at a future time. One may have to go through decades of prevention until the benefits are finally realized.

We are at the start of this book. I know you are excited to get working right away, but we need a few chapters that will set the foundation for your success.

1

WHAT THE BOOK IS ABOUT

"You have your way. I have my way. As for the right way, the correct way, and the only way, it does not exist."
—Friedrich Nietzsche

Every academy, society, college, task force, advisory group, and set of tools has "its way." I have my way, and I will describe it all to you. To be sure, "*the* way" does not exist. Everyone is unique and surrounded by a life of different events with different important details. For the most part, the medical system blends you into a grouped population. In current times we live with task forces, academic panels, and colleges blending you right into the general population. When an organization blends you into the general population, it removes all of your unique aspects. In 2011 the U.S. Preventive Services Task Force (USPSTF) gave recommendations on breast cancer. Aside from causing a massive amount of further confusion, these recommendations did nothing to help prevent breast cancer that spreads.

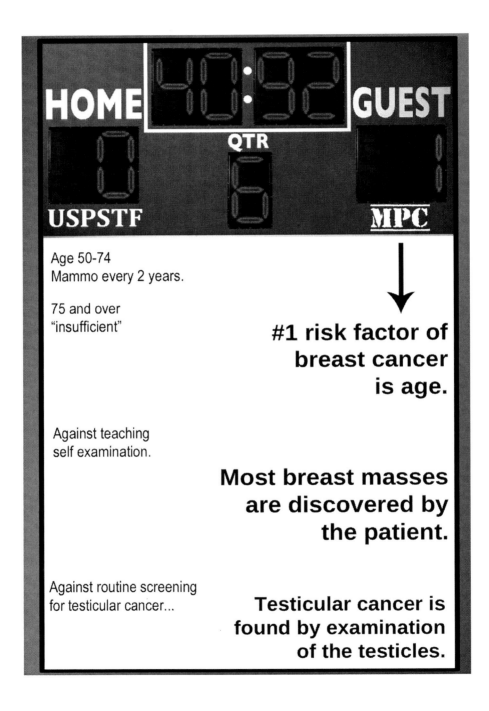

HOME · · GUEST

QTR

USPSTF   MPC

Age 50-74
Mammo every 2 years.

75 and over
"insufficient"

#1 risk factor of breast cancer is age.

Against teaching
self examination.

Most breast masses are discovered by the patient.

Against routine screening
for testicular cancer...

Testicular cancer is found by examination of the testicles.

USPSTF 2011 recommended that women between the ages of fifty and seventy-four have a mammogram every two years. For women over the age of seventy-five, the USPSTF concluded that the current evidence was insufficient to assess benefits and harms.

MEDICAL PREVENTION CENTER—the number one risk factor of breast cancer is age. The USPSTF stated, "No women 75 years or older have been included in the multiple randomized clinical trials of breast cancer screening." The task force also again stated, "Breast cancer is a leading cause of death in older women." The USPSTF recommended against teaching breast self-examination. **MEDICAL PREVENTION CENTER**—the patient discovers most breast masses.

The USPSTF recommended against routine screening for testicular cancer in asymptomatic adolescents.[17] **MEDICAL PREVENTION CENTER**—an exam of the testicles uncovers most testicular cancer.

I will not be kind to task forces that have published guidelines based upon little intelligent thought or simple common sense. You do not need a report to tell you that it hurts when you stub your foot. If you did rely upon a task force for information about stubbing your foot, you would find that because everyone usually recovers and the pain doesn't last, stubbing your foot does not hurt.

CANCERS ARE ASYMPTOMATIC. Cancers are almost always asymptomatic when they are in the early stages. As a cancer advances in size many symptoms could be blamed on noncancer medical conditions. You need to understand that many of the symptoms that a cancer will cause can also be caused by something that is not a cancer. This is part of the reason that many cancers are not detected until they are advanced; you seldom get a distinct warning. Your body doesn't just simply shout out to you that you have a cancer. Please do not start to freak out and think that every single symptom that you have could be related to a cancer. A whole chapter is dedicated to this topic.

DIFFERENT PATH: After over a decade of studying and practicing medicine, I ended up on a totally different path than what is nationally recommended. I take my national boards and remain certified; I do many hours of continuing medical education; and I read daily. I have given you a brief taste of how your medical care may be faulty. But, most important, it's what you are *not* reading that is vital to you. You would have to be dedicated to be a nonmedical person and have a good understanding of current medical thoughts and practices. You cannot only read a study of a new drug or procedure; you also need to pull the references of that study and read them. Authors often boast about their conclusions in a separate work, and unless you read the additional work, you miss these conclusions.

Part of being a physician is the interaction with others who are starting their life in the study of medicine. "Always check the references" is a recurring mantra that the medical students hear from me. Often this statement is used as a teaching point to stress that individuals deserve accuracy of results in their testing. Gone should be the days of "within normal limits," "examination normal," "negative findings," and "you're fine." You deserve to know what is happening on the inside. You deserve to know what a medical study or test gave as a result. When a medical provider has done nothing more than look at you briefly and told you that you are fine, you need to stand up for yourself and be prepared to fight for your medical attention.

This work is not so much a protest against the current state of medical attention in the United States as it is a departure from mainstream thought. Current medicine treats you as a member of a population, and that does not always work when your medical conditions are unique to you. Reflect on the following illustration to understand that although current medicine has developed into many branches, the area of medicine that applies modern science to your needs is missing.

The development of current medicine in the end has taken a confusing and convoluted path. Changes in associations and divisions that happened decades ago still affect how we get our care today. As related to this illustration, I would want you to understand that as current medicine has fractured into so many different specialty and subspecialty areas, there is a lack of Medical Prevention. One need only look to the last two decades of medicine, as there has been an explosion of new subspecialties. Many of the new areas of medicine have given their attention to a narrow range of medical conditions. A division between a physician of medicine and a provider of health care has occurred. Current medicine is often referred to as *evidence-based medicine*. Evidence-based medicine uses algorithms, meta-analysis data, and systematic reviews to influence your medical care. Because of this, most health care teams are unable to respond to you as a unique individual—you are part of the herd. Medical Prevention should stand out as a new area of medicine, or a new basic type of medical philosophy applying current scientific abilities to you as a unique individual to prevent cancer from spreading, to prevent types of sudden death, and to prevent dementia.

1900

Gynecology, OB/GYN 1927

Stomatology 1931

Neurology, Orthopedic Surgery, Pediatrics, Radiology, Urology 1935

General Surgery 1937

Plastic Surgery, Anesthesiology, Craniofacial (Head and Neck), Facial Cosmetic Surgery, Microsurgery, Craniomaxillofacial Trauma, Cosmetic Surgery 1941

Physical Medicine and Rehabilitation 1947

Preventitive Medicine, Proctology, Colorectal Surgery 1949

Family Medicine, Cardiology 1969

Gastroenterology, Cardiovascular Surgery, Thoracic Surgery, Rhumatology, Nephrology, Hematology, Infectious Disease, Allergy and Immunology, Endocrinology 1971

Fertility Medicine, Maternal-Fetal Medicine, Oncology, Internal Medicine, Reproductive Medicine Dermatopathology, Pediactic Nephrology, Pediatric Oncology, Pediatric Surgery 1973

Emergency Medicine 1979

Early Medicine- ↑
(more medicine— less health-care)

Geriatric Medicine, Critical Care Medicine, Surgical Critical Care, Trauma Care, Pediatric Critical Care Medicine, Geriatric Medicine 1985

Pediatric and Adolescent Gyn 1987

Geriatric Psychiatry, Preventive Medicine Undersea, Pathology-Pediatric, Sports Medicine, Clinical Cardiac Electrophisiology 1989

Adolescent Medicine, Pediatric Emergency Medicine, Medical Research Genetics, Pain Medicine, Pain Management, Addiction Psychiatry, Pediatrice Infectious Disease, Nutrition Specalists 1991

Vascular Neurology, Pediatric Radiology, Vascular and Interventional Radilogy 1993

Spinal Cord Injury Medicine 1995

Developmental-behavioral Pediatrics, Molecular Genetic Pathology, Interventional Cardiology, Child Psychiatry, Pediatric Rehabilitation Medicine, Neurodevelopmental Disabilities 1999

Musculoskeletal Oncology 2001

Disaster Medicine, Psychosomatic Medicine, Foot and Ankle, Surgical Sports Medicine, Hepatology 2003

Sleep Specialty, Pain Medicine, Sleep Medicine, Neuromuscular Medicine 2005

Thoracic Surgery-congenital Cardiac Surgery, Medical Biochemical Genetics, Cardiothoracic 2007

Urgent Care Medicine 2009

Female Pelvic Medicine and Reconstructive Surgery, Critical Care ER Medicine, Complex General Surgical Oncology, Cardiovascular Disease, Oncologic Sugery, Brain Injury Medicine, Clinical Informatics, Sleep Medicine 2011

Androcology (Future)

2020

Forensic Medicine 1900
Ophthalmology 1916
Otolaryngology, or ENT 1924
Endocrinology 1930
Dermatology 1932
Cellular Pathology, Pathology 1936

Infectious Disease 1940
Maxillofacial Surgery 1945

Clinical Chemistry, Pulmonology, Nephrology 1950
Pediatric Nephrology, Pediatric Endocrinology 1960
Clinical Laboratory Sciences 1968
MOHS Surgery, Pulmonary Disease 1970

Nuclear Radiology, Child and Adolescent Psychiatry, Neurosurgery, Medical Oncology, Blood Banking/Transfusion, Pediatric Cardiology 1972
Neonatal Intensive Care 1974
Pediatric Endocrinology 1976

Rheumatology, Geriatrics, Pediatric Hematology 1980

Current Medicine
(less medicine—more health-care)

Spine Specialty, Pediatric Pulmonary 1984

Hand Surgery, Intensive Care, Adolescent Gynecology, Pediatric Infectious Disease 1986

Clinical Microbiology, Clinical Immunology, Cytopathology, P Gi 1988

Clinical Neurophysiology, Pediatric Orthopedic Surgery, Pediatric Rhumatology, Neuropsychiatry, Vascular Surgery 1990

Forensic Psychiatry, Medical Toxicology, Sports Medicine, Adolescent Medicine, Neurotology, Pediatric Otolaryngology 1992

Neuroradiology 1994
Interventional Cardiology 1996
Pain Medicine 1998

Pediatric Dermatology, Undersea and Hyperbaric Medicine, Adolescent Medicine, Bariatric Surgery, Head and Neck, Facial Cosmetic Surgery, Craniofacial Surgery 2000

Hospice and Palliative Medicine, Palliative Care, Child Abuse Pediatrics, Sports Medicine, Pediatric Urology 2006

Advanced Heart Failure and Transplant Cardiology 2008
Pediatric Transplant Hepatology 2009

Emergency Medical Services 2010

Medical Prevention 2012

Medical Prevention

An area of medicine that combines different concepts into a philosophy of medical care. This new area of medicine applies the science of medicine to the motivated unique individual. Working at the level of the individual to detail prevention of disease states, medical prevention does not apply general guidelines that cover large populations.

Medical Prevention has been almost totally missed. This book calls for a new way of thinking about medicine and science. The truth is that most people do not care about their own health. Few people feel personally responsible for their medical conditions; however, some want proper attention to details. Many just take whatever comes their way, and when something bad happens, they wish they had done more. When something bad happens, they want more options. It is all about the attention to the prevention—Medical Prevention.

One can prevent types of sudden death by being aware of the conditions before they result in catastrophe. One can prevent dementia by mitigation of the causes. (Some of the information provided here can be considered controversial, as new medical concepts will need years to develop.) Much of the dementia prevention work is based upon hypothesis: *The Micron Stroke Hypothesis of Alzheimer's Disease and Dementia.*[18]

The consequences of some medical conditions are so severe that they need to be taken very seriously *even if there is only a very small chance that they could exist.*

This is not a "cup of lavender tea" to help you get through life unharmed. This book doesn't tell you what type of herb you should take for a specific medical problem. It's not a way for you to lose weight, and it's not a polemic against corporate control, malfeasance, and systemic corruption (I have strong feelings about those things, but airing them is not my purpose here). This book is a road map and a tool for you to use in protecting yourself and your loved ones. It's not a solution to the corruption of the CDC, the FDA, or the government. Yes, I suspect there is some corruption in the branches of the government that are able to control such huge swings of corporate market shares with a single statement or announcement. This is not to be a stomping ground for corporations and malfeasance that they commit or some magical revelations into their corporate corruption. Plain and simple: corporations want to make money. You are just a line on the balance sheet—understand and respect that fact. Don't expect to change all of it. Let us move forward.

**"Do not pray for easy lives. Pray to be stronger men."
—Phillips Brooks and then John F. Kennedy**

You go to the doctor and are told what you can do and cannot do based upon your insurance. That is just not good enough! You deserve to know what you can do and cannot do, and not have your doctor cutting you off and preventing you from taking care of yourself. You are going through a psychological abandonment from your health care provider.

For some this book is not going to pay off for years. The benefit of doing prevention is something like that of wearing a seat belt in an automobile: you can put on a seat belt every time get into a car, yet it might not be for years and years until there is a time that the belt saves you. For many who are reading this book, prevention is the same way. You take certain actions year after year in the interest of prevention. You might wait a decade until you reap the harvest of your prevention. I will say, however, that on that day you will be very happy you were doing what you needed to do to take care of yourself or your loved ones.

Information about specific disease states and how they develop and progress is available in many other publications. When needed, I will supply basic information so you can stay with me. The intention of the book is not to be a primer on specific disease states. The book covers only what you need to know about and how to avoid—common cancers that spread, sudden death, and dementia. For detailed information on certain medical conditions, seek out additional reading on your own.

Imagine the enormous complexity of building an aircraft carrier. Thousands of hours of planning and teamwork are required to carry out the specific details—yet aircraft carriers are built. Although we can and do accomplish similarly complex tasks when it comes to fighting diseases in some cases, often—and for a variety of reasons—we simply don't. If you were to ask current medicine to build an aircraft carrier, chances are you would end up with ... well, I will let your own experience with current medicine fill in what type of boat you would end up with and whether it would float. (I take a moment here to explain that I am not disappointed in all of medicine. Oftentimes a health care team is top-notch for the conditions that it treats. Members of the team are caring and appropriate. Lives are saved because of skilled people performing important procedures. Not everything in current medicine is broken. Some aspects are functioning perfectly, and people do sometimes get the care that they need. I just want to be clear that I am telling you we can do better. We should no longer have the laziness of health-care teams who are guided by insurance company restrictions and faulty guidelines. I am confident that for every "amazing" outcome you know of, there are multiple times when the health care system lets you down).

I have reviewed and integrated the data and conclusions from some of the largest clinical trials and landmark medical studies into this book. I spared no trees in the preparation of the endnotes for this book. I evaluated and reviewed hundreds of articles.

An important part of this book is explaining how you as an individual should have your own guide—*How to take care of yourself and prevent cancers that are easily preventable.* The general population following current guidelines will end up going through their lives discovering that they have actually developed certain diseases. Current guidelines anticipate the diseases—yet do little to prevent them.

The plan in this book will not save everyone. This is not an answer to world health care. This is not an answer to government health care or any issue that involves politics. This book outlines what *you need to do,* with the direct thoughts, scientific data, and literature to support that approach. This is a guide to take you step by step through many of the medical conditions you might have or might develop, the majority of which your health care team and your doctor will never discover. In the final chapter, "What Else Can Be Done?" I provide a step-by-step example for those who read the rest of this work but do not discover what they need to consider about their own body.

Preventive health is a popular term, but the health care system does not do it. Preventive health from your medical provider is limited to what an insurance company will cover or pay for. There are some rare examples of genetic testing that some companies offer, but the results probably don't change your individual plan. A physician is unable to do proper prevention because he will be at risk of noncompliance with the insurance company. Testing is often necessary but is not covered by insurance. When can the doctor be "the doctor" and tell you what you need, not what your insurance will cover or pay for? This is the root of the current state of psychological abandonment of your health care team. Your doctor is unable to give you the advice you need because, like all other providers, she has agreed to just go with the flow and do only what the insurance company and guidelines tell her to do or not do. In this setting you no longer need that health care provider. Google could provide your medical care better than a provider can who is just spoon-feeding you guidelines designed by politics. If you don't believe what I am telling you, continue to read. I will take apart the guidelines for you so you can see that following your current path there is no way your first stroke is going to be prevented or your ovarian cancer will be detected before it spreads or that you can prevent Alzheimer's dementia. Read on and you will have answers.

When you have a medical problem, you need to have some independent opinions. People need to fight for their health care more often. There is a battle going on against your insurance company or HMO. These companies are trying to contain costs (make more profits) and grade doctors (based on how much money they spend). Some aspects of this are good, but others are just tools used to shift blame and make it look as though they have reasons to take such huge profits. World leaders have publicly spoken on this subject,[19] yet no significant change happens. This is why *you* need to know what to do. No one will help you. You are alone. You need to be vigilant!

Hypothesis: "The history of medicine over the last thirty years has developed and splintered into so many subspecialty components that an aspect of true Medical Prevention has been overlooked." —Allen J. Orehek, MD

After you've completed this book, I hope you will agree. In the early writing of this book, a member of a focus group commented that medicine has been "divided and conquered." I agree with her totally. Reflecting on the time line on page 7, you will notice how for decades the "doctor has been out."

This book sets the framework for a new line of doctors: Medical Prevention specialists. (Not preventive specialists as indicated by the American Board of Specialists). These new doctors will not need to base their recommendations and plans based upon the whims of the bottom line of an insurance company. These physicians will be able to apply current science to a unique individual, not guidelines to groups of people. This group of real doctors will be back to the profession of medicine, only to be distained by other doctors who are stuck in the profession of health care. The return of the physician of medicine to whom you trust your medical problems can work side by side with a doctor who provides health care.

2

WHO THE BOOK IS FOR

This book is for you if you do not worry about money but do worry about developing diseases such as Alzheimer's. Proper prevention of dementia means being evaluated according to the *science* of the disease, not the health care aspects of it. Prevention of dementia would overwhelm any current health care team, but you should be informed of a choice. It is your brain at stake.

This book is for you if you worry about developing cancers that could spread and want to know what you could do before they spread in your body.

Read this book if you want to prevent a death from cancer.

Read this book if you or anyone you know wants to prevent Alzheimer's dementia.

This book is for you if you are interested in the diseases that affect the baby boomers. Large sums of money are spent on treatment of preventable disorders such as strokes, Alzheimer's, and dementia.

If you agree with the proposition "we do not know it all," then you should continue to read this book. Imagine a pool of water with no waves. The surface is perfectly still. See the reflection of light on the glass-like surface.

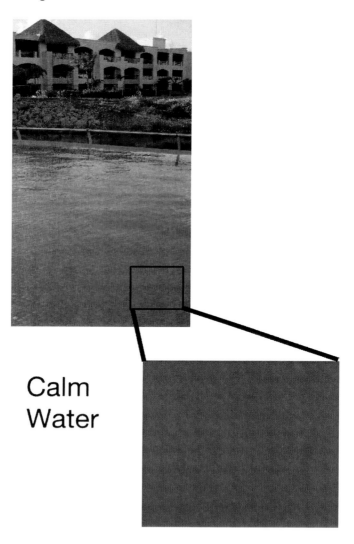

Calm
Water

Now imagine splashing the surface slightly and making a wave. See how the wave of water goes to the edges of the pool and then reflects back toward the middle. Watch how one wave interacts with another wave. Waves grow and fall as they combine and clash with other waves. As you recall the first wave, I am sure you were able to predict with general accuracy when it would impact the edge of the pool. This is because the brain allows you to make such a prediction based upon laws of nature.

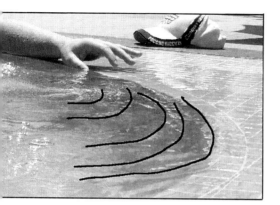

Splash

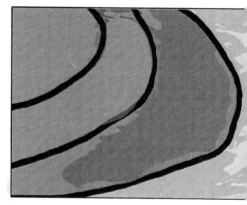

Consider that even with all of the power of your brain, you might not understand much at all. A full release of intellectual power would allow you to predict what the surface of the pool looks like after five minutes. Perhaps a computer model would be able to simulate and get the answer correct. Perhaps someone with some good luck at guessing would get it correct. Most people might agree with me that picking what the correct wave pattern would be after minutes of wave-on-wave interaction would be difficult or even impossible.

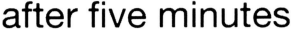

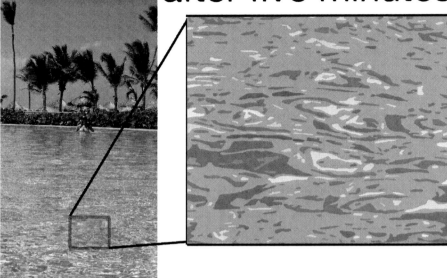

This book is not for the person who cannot appreciate that there are factors interacting with each other that are quite impossible to predict. In much the same way, some aspects of disease interactions are out of the reach of our understanding. Some factors are difficult to prove in some settings. Some aspects of disease prevention reveal new, unique aspects of your body, and they require additional detailed thought in considering.

This book will save your life or the life of someone you hold dear (or you are investing a lot of money in). Companies and private corporations invest millions in an individual person yet never know what that person is really made of inside. This book will allow you to mitigate the risks of many disease problems that will strike without warning.

Keep reading if you hire or manage an elite workforce. You want healthy and resilient people staffing your important posts, don't you? This book will help you to preserve the people valuable to you. It is understood that your motivations are in protecting your investment. Imagine protecting your human investment right alongside every piece of equipment that you also own. Your company would never purchase a piece of equipment without some type of warranty or inspection, verifying that parts and components are operating properly. Why then would you or your company invest in an individual without doing the same minimum evaluation? When a Ferrari is made in the factory, one of the stages in its production is to check for any defects. The automobile is checked at eight hundred separate points on the frame, simply for alignment. All the other components go through additional checks, but the frame gets checked in eight hundred separate locations. Why is it that a human body is not taken care of with the same intensity?

To fully understand this work, you need to realize that what you hold in your hands is the advice that comes to *you* as a unique *individual*. Few components of this book are designed to be simply rubber-stamped across large populations. Perhaps in an additional work, adjustments could be directed toward en masse treatment; but this work is for you. You may find this point simple, but treating you as a unique individual through every step of your medical care differs greatly from treating you as part of a group of population. If you do not agree, then perhaps reading this book will not be the best use of your time.

If you find interest in this next short section, then this book is for you.

John Ritter died at age fifty-four from a rupture of his thoracic aorta (the "water main" that exits the heart and the largest artery in the body). A simple ultrasound of that structure could have detected the flaw years before it ruptured. I have detected many aortic enlargements and aneurysms in patients over the years. Many have undergone surgery and gone on to live normal lives. Many are observed over time for changes. Some shrink a bit with medications and medical treatment. John Ritter died hours after the onset of his symptoms. Often people who have this problem find out only when they fall over; at this point, there's only a slight chance they will be alive after an operation. I challenge you to consider the condition of your aorta: is it enlarged? Your doctor will tell you "it's fine" until you have it evaluated or develop a problem. You will have no symptoms until you fall over and require an emergency operation.

Why have you not had an ultrasound of your heart? We agree that your heart is one of the most important organs you have, so why do you not give it any attention? These questions are just to get you thinking about how far behind you could really be when it comes to your body.

Someone should have told Patrick Swayze, who died from pancreatic cancer, that an MRI of the pancreas every few years could have picked up his problem as treatable and curable.[20] Famous actors who suffer from miscarriages might have some beautiful kids running around.[21] All the money and fame does not get them proper advice to care for their bodies properly. No guidelines direct a health care team to do such a detailed workup when a woman has multiple miscarriages. If physicians simply knew enough to do a detailed hypercoagulable state workup on someone with multiple miscarriages, it would be the first step to treating that patient properly. Many high-risk obstetricians and hematologists understand how to treat a patient with miscarriages once they are given the diagnosis—a factor deficiency or similar problem. I have half a dozen children who are my patients whose mothers, when they came to me, had multiple miscarriages and were unable to get pregnant. The diagnosis was relatively simple, and it's often overlooked because it doesn't appear on any thorough and complete guideline of what to do when a woman has miscarriages.[i]

---

i   Some general guidelines exist for miscarriages; however, they do not include the **MPC** hypercoagulable state evaluation.

3

WHO THE BOOK IS NOT FOR

If you are looking for some rare herb, special medicine, or other quick fix, then this book is not for you. Science, proof, data, experience, and common sense are the ingredients that go into your recipe for cure. The cure is possible—prevention is difficult. Acupuncture, yoga, meditation, and other behaviors fit in nicely with what I am explaining. Realize that nothing is a quick fix. You cannot cheat nature. Prevention is complicated and difficult. (But you can do it!) Medical Prevention is a lifestyle.

This book is not for someone who wants to debate the long history of statin medications *without* digging into the real facts and data. You can find answers to your fears when you slow down a bit and look at all of the details as they relate to a specific product. You could be a unique person for whom such medications cause side effects—however, you also could have a misplaced fear. As a great movie you just watched is not the same as the last movie you enjoyed—not all statin medications are the same. There are many statin products I would not give to a dog—they do not work effectively enough for my patients' goals—and they have too many side effects. You do need to find your place in this great debate, as this is a class of drugs and each is different.

If you succumb to stress and anxiety easily or don't see the value in hard work, this book is not for you. Medical Prevention requires vigilance, patience, and the constitution to embrace intimidating knowledge and therapies. When a dentist read the manuscript, he added here that at times the cure could be worse than the disease. Those who cannot deal with tension and anxiety may find the path to prevention a bit longer and rougher. For some anything new or unknown adds anxiety and stress—so medical prevention is simply another typical day.

Those who are living in poverty—40 million in the United States—will have an even larger challenge requiring exceptional focus, energy, and time to participate in the benefits of Medical Prevention. People who have just lost their jobs because of the economy and have no medical insurance and people who are struggling to put food on the table to pay their bills that were due months ago will note similar obstacles. If you are looking at foreclosure on your home, then this is not going to be a time in your life to get started with any significant aspect of the medical attention that you need. This book is not for you if you are dealing with significant medical problems already. If your genetic code has given you many problems that will consume most of your "doctoring" time, then you may not benefit from all of this—unless you are dedicated. If you are dedicated, then you might be able to complete all of the tasks necessary to care for your existing medical conditions and the additional work necessary to prevent others.

Using Medical Prevention to take care of your body is not easy—it requires work. You have to arrange and coordinate a good deal of information. The information needs to be evaluated for accuracy and applied to your unique situation. Gathering stacks of information that lack proper quality and details will simply have you stumbling. Production of quality reports in health care is rare—as there are few standards. This book is an introduction to a trillion-dollar industry. The prevention of medical conditions is just at the genesis of creation. We are in the Stone Age, or whatever prehistoric time was before that. Paul Dudley White, MD, president of the American Heart Association in 1941, once described the early years as a time of "almost unbelievable ignorance" about heart disease.[22] I would say that we currently have an almost unbelievable ignorance about Medical Prevention. Circumstances could change, and I do have hope.

This book is not for you if you are covered by a traditional health plan (no matter how good you think it is) or if you are getting your care from a doctor who follows all the guidelines *and of whom you never ask any questions*. However, if you use this book to ask proper questions, you could still benefit from the results. This book is not 100 percent perfect. It's like a piece of world-class software from a major operating system vendor that often has bugs that need to be worked out—system freezes, memory leaks, and other problems. Nothing seems to be perfect; there are many ways to complete the same task. My work here with you is to improve your understanding of what you need to be looking for in your medical attention. The goal is not for 100 percent perfection but simply to do better than you currently are.

I would not at all be surprised if after you had contact with the **MEDICAL PREVENTION CENTER** and received your "homework" assignment that you started to cry. So many people have no clue as to what is happening with their own bodies. Many people feel uneasy and get the feeling that they could already be too late in discovering what is happening inside their bodies. If you are someone who gets anxious thinking about things you should be doing but aren't, then perhaps this work is not for you.

This book is not for you if you believe that once symptoms start, you have enough time to resolve a medical condition. You must understand that *now* is the time to discover what is going on with your body so you can prevent problems.

This work does not provide information about declarative memory, procedural memory, or other categories of memory. If you want to have a better understanding of different types of memory, then a different resource would be better for you. After completing research on my *Micron Stroke Hypothesis of Alzheimer's Disease and Dementia*, I realized how little we understand the working of the brain. Despite decades of research, very little about the brain is completely understood. Medical science has only scratched the surface of what your brain is able to do, so much more is hidden from our understanding. If you are looking for specific examples and detailed explanations of such topics, you will need a different reference. Volumes have been written on different types of memory, and a neuropsychologist will bend your ear explaining how little we really understand in the functioning of our consciousness.

I am not writing about quality-adjusted life years lost or gained. I will leave this interpretation to the analysis that is part of prospective studies. If you want to read a resource that puts people into an equation, then you will not find this book much help. *I have yet to meet anyone who fits into an equation—they find it very uncomfortable!* Everyone is unique. You have had a unique life, and the events that surround you are not the same for the person next to you.

If you have all of your faith in your personal health insurance company, then this book is not for you. Understand that corporations' main idea is in making money, and we simply exist as only pixels and dots on their bottom line. As Eckhart Tolle said, "You do not actually matter to corporations at all."[23] These would be the insurance companies that just make money without providing the actual care they should. As long as such corporations dictate the standards of care, you will never get any of the care you really need. If you are the owner or CEO of a large health care business, then this book is for you—realizing that you will likely use the information for your personal health, but no way will the subscribers to your plan get this attention and prevention. I agree that Medical Prevention could overwhelm a health care team, given the current system design.

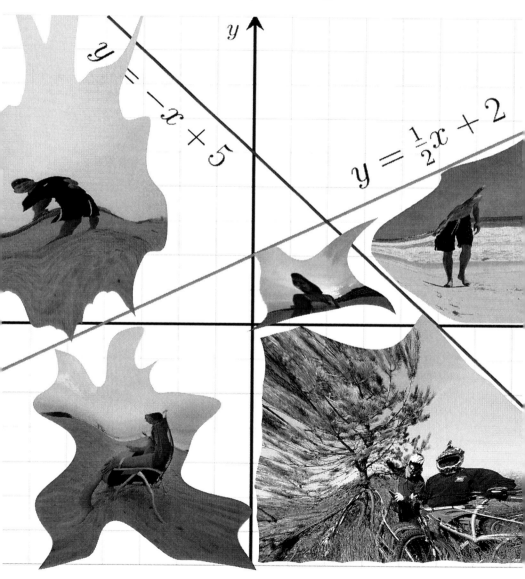

When you are the "loved one," not taking care of your body is actually selfish. Your neglect can lead to significant pain and suffering to others around you. You are not the one who will drive to the nursing or personal care home after work every day to visit. You are not the one who will have to look on as a loved one dies from metastatic breast cancer. You are not the one who will be talking with hospice nurses as plans are made for pain control of a cancer that has spread. You are not the one who will have to provide constant reorientation to the demented loved one. You are not the one who will go and have a good cry every time that a grandchild asks, "What is wrong with Grandma?" You are the selfish loved one who let dementia take hold. You *are* the one who is not doing what you should do to prevent these events from happening.

Finally, this is not a book that tries to stir up controversy over vitamin D. Years ago when vitamin D literature caught my eye, I integrated it into my medical practice. I was surprised that the majority of patients that wanted to be checked—from a seven-year-old boy to a twenty-five-year-old girl who is a sun worshiper to all of the aged—had low vitamin D levels. I don't think this is a new medical situation, but we have now identified it, and it deserves attention. In my part of the country, everyone has a low vitamin D level until proven that they have a normal one. I am positive vitamin D is important, but what diseases and cures can be related to this vitamin is still under scientific evaluation.

4

ARE DOCTORS MUDDLED?

How a doctor gets accurate and correct information is a complex problem. There are many basic physiological subjects and anatomy, things that do not change often, but most of what a doctor needs to pay attention to is how the influence of current literature changes the aspects of medicine and medical care. Your health care team can be behind the times not because of laziness, but because often some of the information that is provided comes from questionable sources. When a source of information is based upon weak data, confused data, erroneous conclusions, or inaccurate results, then that is a weak and questionable source, regardless of the name stamped on the paper. Your doctor is pummeled daily by insurance companies, private companies, drug and technology companies, task force recommendations, and other ventures that want your doctor to follow their agenda. There is no doubt that the publicity of meta-analysis reports changes the practice of your doctor. Your doctor might not be lazy, but when the decisions of your health care provider are based on junk science, well, you get junk medical advice.

Alternatively, your health care provider can be surrounded by science, physiology, common sense, good scientific data, and experience in the art of medicine. Your doctor is either a system doctor who is simply standing in line ready to give you your "fast food"-style medical care, based upon the newest plans from the insurance companies and the meta-analysis reports, or your provider is a "real doc—physician of medicine." Using this book will help you to decide what type of medical care you are getting and how to ask for more detailed answers. Your mind will start to wonder if you are getting medical care or health care.

To understand what the term *doctors* means, we need to look at what functions doctors perform. First, let's examine the number of doctors in the United States. From the total number of medical doctors you need to remove those who do not provide face-to-face or direct medical care to patients. They work for insurance companies, perform research or administrative duties, or are retired. Now, remove the doctors who are not involved with primary contact with patients in an outpatient setting (where prevention should happen). Remove all of the specialists who are deeply accurate in their field but have a challenge linking diseases from different organ systems. You are left with a list of doctors who are in the specialties of pediatrics, internal medicine, family medicine, and internal medicine/pediatrics. From those, you have to remove the doctors who have psychologically abandoned their patients. You need to remove most of the employed docs who have to follow the rules of their boss. Employed doctors often face a penalty if they refer out of the system. Because of formulary limitations, they have to follow ever-changing restrictions on what drugs they can advise. The employed doctors also have to tolerate passing along substandard recommendations to avoid insurance obstacles or administrative hassles. Some of these doctors are even penalized when they step out of the box. Many of these are "system doctors—providers of health care," at times placed into a health care insurance empire. The employed "system doctor" works to restrain costs and testing. Profits from rationing of your health care then go back to that insurance company. As we work closer to that small inner circle of "real doctors," you find many doctors out of touch with current data. They need additional help and support. Finally, we arrive at the innermost circles, and this is what is left for taking care of you. In the United States, this is a small group. These real doctors base their treatment plans upon science, physiology, anatomy, data, experience, art of medicine, and common sense.

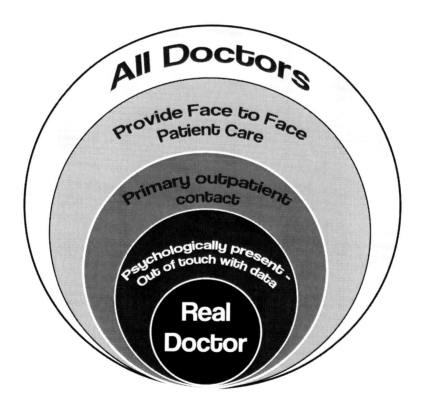

Missing a correct diagnosis is not always the doctor's fault. Some diagnoses are extremely rare or difficult to make. Doctors face legal action when a missed diagnosis results in a poor outcome. The United States has no check or balance to prevent doctors from being tortured with legal problems in the face of rare problems. The other side of this coin is that many doctors simply never convey that they do not know. I find it rare that a doctor tells the patient that he doesn't know the answer but will call in a specialist or consult literature or read more on the subject. "I don't know" are powerful words, and often what follows is an improvement in the patient care—doctors want to help fix you up. No one can know it all. Often when one does not know, the next step is to ask questions. Questions can be your friend as you fight for your medical and health care. Questions can improve the quality of your health care. Doctors agree that they are often not able to care for their patients the way they really wish they could.[ii]

How did doctors get so far away from the science and medicine that used to be at the heart of the profession? What happened is a toxic concoction of pressures from nonmedical agendas. The list of ingredients for this chemical spill includes legal concerns, insurance company profits, malpractice worries, doctor and provider training by a less-than-accurate system, cost-based task forces, understudied advances in medicine, the simple breadth of medicine, psychological abandonment of patients, and so on. We have bred many providers of health care and neglected physicians of medicine.

When you want to communicate in medicine, often you must use an entirely different language. The terminology and abbreviations are all new to a medical student. A common problem today is moving medical and scientific language forward while allowing the common lexicon to catch up. Many people on the street know what a blood clot or pulmonary embolism is. Once a medical term is rooted into the common language, the term no longer evolves or refines easily. Often people in the medical field then start to make charts or break down terms into classes or categories, further complicating subjects that are not well understood to start with. A common myth is that Eskimos have many different words for snow. Although it's false, in this case

---

ii   A difference between medical care and health care.

you can imagine how useful it might be to have several words for what may seem like a single thing. The same is true for medicine, where an expanded vocabulary is hugely advantageous. Often in medicine we need to describe a dozen different degrees of a disorder, yet all we are left with is "mild," "moderate," and "severe." Also, medicine has always struggled with developing proper terminology as new discoveries are made. Our language lets us down.

Even doctors are confused as to how to care for themselves. They are not lazy, but they might catch CNN or the *U.S. News & World Report* rather than read the articles and look at the data. The things I hated about residency and medical school were journal club and literature reviews. I hated these mostly because I was often assigned subject matter that I had no interest in or I had to listen to someone speak on a topic that I had no interest in. I found that as a private physician I spend most of my time reviewing articles and scientific data. Often, I not only review the new data but also end up reading the references that the authors cite. Published articles can be difficult to get through. Correctly interpreting medical literature to use it as a reference is a difficult task because often the reference itself has its own multiple references. Much work is needed to read all of the data and verify its integrity. From how the researchers design the study to how they collect the data to how they interpret the results—even landmark studies have glaring faults and incorrect conclusions. (I go into detail in a later section as I walk you through a major medical literature publication that cost a company hundreds of millions of dollars. Yes, even companies that own multibillion-dollar drugs make errors in how they publish and collect data. I will walk you through a landmark medical study and explain to you clearly the inaccurate conclusions.)

Even a good doctor can be thrown off his proper course by the results of testing that he ordered unless he is prepared to look at the data and sort through the results. I ask you, how do you feel the day before a stroke? How do you feel and act the day before a massive myocardial infarction? How do you feel and act a week before you learn you have metastatic cancer? For the most part, no symptoms come from your disease, that is until it's usually too late.

5

CURRENT MEDICINE: THE DOCTOR IS OUT

My experience as a physician is different from that of many other physicians because as a solo physician I never had to work within the restrictions/guidelines of health maintenance organizations and the brutalities of insurance company guidelines and restrictions of care. I recall one time being on the phone when my patient was in the intensive care unit (ICU), and the insurance carrier called to let me know it had approved the case for another day of ICU care. I said, "Good thing because he has a tube coming out of his mouth allowing him to breath!"

I am able to give people medical advice based on current scientific literature, common sense, science, and my own experience. Unlike many physician friends of mine who essentially hate their lives and the places they work—I am able to get up every day with an awesome amount of energy, looking forward to seeing and treating people based on their specific needs. Patients should be treated as unique individuals based on the current trends in medical science, technology, and medications. I have often told people that if they hit the lottery while in my parking lot and come back to see me saying, "Hey, doc, I'm rich now. What can I do to take care of myself?" my response would be the same: "Do exactly what I've been telling you to do." I will share with you the same details that you need to develop the proper understanding of what your body needs. Every car that comes off the lot has had its brakes checked before you drive it, yet often even the simple things that we can do to help understand our own bodies are never part of our health care team's plan.

Medicine and health care are often used interchangeably. When you seek attention for health problems or medical concerns you are not sure if the advice you receive comes from a branch of medicine or from health care. Medicine, as you understand it, should represent a constant progression of the art of healing and science of diseases. Health care is the card that you have in your pocket that allows you access to medicine. Many doctors agree with me that currently those two have been blended so closely into one that when you seek medical attention, you get mostly health care. You and I could chat for hours about this topic, all I need is for you to consider the difference.

I wrote already about employed doctors. I am sure there are rare cases of employed doctors treating people exactly as they should be treated; however, it usually does not last. Most often the employed docs have their eyes glazed over. They gave up by signing a contract. They provide care and make a profit for their boss. I am sure they have to tell themselves good things at night so they can sleep. They know that they traded any political fight for patient care by simply going with the rest of the crowd. They have to stay on formulary (list of drugs that you or your doctor can pick from that your insurance company has approved) or get a pay cut. They allow the insurance company to decide what drugs you are qualified for. They order testing based upon what your insurance guidelines call for. This leaves you with a ton of robots. You would be better off with a computer program making the decisions based upon data that you put into the blank boxes.

Hospital time is a difficult problem. You might not be admitted because your insurance company denies coverage. Your doctor might want you in the hospital, but she is not able to do it at times because of insurance restraints. Often a patient is sent home from the emergency room only to go out into the parking lot and have a catastrophic event. At times people make it home to then have a disastrous event. This happens because patients are sent home too soon. This also happens because patients are not readmitted because of financial considerations.[24] [25] Most of the population of the United States should prepare for this next decade of care with new rules that will limit your doctor's ability to admit you into the hospital based upon whether you were there over the previous thirty days.[iii]

The medical literature that doctors use in treating your conditions, preventing your illnesses, and advising you on risk reductions comes from a few different sources. The sources of medical literature are unique and range from basic science to complicated reviews that are not easy to understand. On the most essential level, you will have information that is related to basic scientific information—anatomy, physiology, drug pharmacokinetics, and such.

---

iii   With the hospital's not being paid for a readmission, we might agree there will be fewer readmissions—but that will not help you if you are sick and need to be readmitted.

Often the information that comes from these scientific areas changes slowly as advances are proven with animal models and better testing in lab environments. No doubt, significant subdivisions of each of these areas of science exist and have a cumulative effect on the data that is produced with each new understanding. One can consider these areas of science the "best truth" that your health care provider considers when advising you. Confusing the issue is that often the science is difficult to apply in a meaningful way to your current medical situation. So this leaves you with the best type of data available and no easy way to apply them to your medical conditions. So what happens from there?

The next source of data is from medical and scientific literature. Studies are published and examined in a variety of journals and online publications. Some of these studies are complete and thorough. Others are superficial and designed to serve a specific purpose—providing the conclusion the authors wanted.[26] (It is a cynical statement, but the reference backs it up.) Your health care team needs to dig through all of the different articles that are produced each year—a daunting task. For many doctors, sorting through all of that data is simply impossible, so they rely upon guidelines. Once you begin to follow only guidelines, you have taken a large step away from the basic science that is your "best truth" of medical decision making. Rarely do authors who have done a complete and thorough evaluation of all of the data for that subject construct guidelines. When a comprehensive guideline such as this is created, doctors could benefit from following it because they now do not have to dig through all of the different articles[iv]. A good doctor is able to give patients medical advice based on multiple factors that often are unavailable to most health care teams. Most advice that

---

iv   The Medical Prevention Center is looking for guidelines that you may have worked on that fit into this category. If you were an author on a set of guidelines and believe they match the philosophy of this work, please notify us immediately at info at medicalpreventioncenter.com.

I give I base upon current scientific literature (and we have to dig through that to see what is good science and what is junk science), common sense, science, anatomy, histology, physiology, drug pharmacokinetics (how a drug works), local patterns, unique aspects of the patient, and my own experience. Understanding the patient as a unique person allows me to apply many current medical treatments, medications, therapies, technologies, and all else that is the good part of modern medical science.

The remaining data come from all remaining sources: headlines, guidelines, academy recommendations, and meta-analysis data. Although the titles of such produced data sound official, the conclusions and recommendations are often shady. Next time you are getting guidance from your health care team, ask them, "So from what data do you develop this treatment plan?" I would imagine that you get a bunch of stumbling words, an answer different from the last time you asked the same question, or an explanation that it is merely that doctor's "gestalt." Once you know where the advice is generated, you will then be able to make an informed decision of whether that advice is good for you.

When one wants to understand how to develop a treatment plan based upon data/testing, one must understand how all of the data are collected. Think of it in this way: when you want to make a batch of corn muffins, there is never simply one fast step. True, making muffins is a simple thing, but it requires that you put together many smaller steps. The list of ingredients must be accurate. The condition of the ingredients must be proper. The temperature of the oven is important, as is the order in which you combine the ingredients. If you overbeat the batter or cook it at the wrong temperature, you fail, and you won't end up with a perfect crown on the muffins. If you let the batter rest before you cook it, you will have maximum crown on your muffins. (Then you have the best muffin tops!) A similar example is building a home. In building a home, you start with your thoughts of a building. You draw and make sketches that become plans. Then you start building with an integration of subcontractors who need to do their jobs properly if the final building is to be a success. When one contractor doesn't use the properly listed materials, it affects other parts of the building, or a flaw could go unnoticed until a future date when it then becomes a problem. Both of these examples show you how long a process could be and that, for the results to be a success, you need to have all of the little steps completed perfectly.

When you go through medical testing, many parts of the test need to come together even *before* you go for the test. I can tell you that testing at some locations will give you poor, inaccurate, or incomplete results long before you schedule your test there. The reason is that the people at the location gave inaccurate, incomplete, or superficial results in the past as part of their general operating philosophy. If they had provided inaccurate results in the past over and over, what would make you think that you would be able to get accurate results this time around? Yes, most of these places have all of the proper certification from the state or federal government. They have "qualified" individuals who either do your work and mess it up or do their part properly only to have someone in the next step mess it up. When there are so many different steps involved in data/testing, it is easy for any one of the steps to occur improperly and end up giving you inaccurate results. Appreciate how difficult it is to get all of the proper details of each step lined up perfectly for an accurate result. Simply understanding this fact will help you with your medical conditions by understanding that nothing is perfectly accurate. People can improve the accuracy of their results when they obtain additional opinions of data/testing.

When you need to go for a medical test that includes many substeps, remember that the results may not be 100 percent accurate.

It is beyond this book to explain all of the different basic types of studies and how they are designed and carried out. For a more complete idea, consult randomized clinical trials, cohort studies, case series, case-controlled series, observational studies, clinical investigations, systematic reviews, animal research, laboratory studies, case reports, and meta-analyses. From this list you can understand how difficult it is for your health care team to try to get you the right data for your problem. The body is exceedingly complex. So remember, when you see on TV or the news that a new study is released with some flashy headline, be sure to consider how the study was designed. Knowing where your data come from helps you to decide whether to use it or observe it.

In the United States, preventive medicine—one among dozens of recognized medical specialties—is represented by The American Board of Preventive Medicine. Started in 1948, this division of medicine, to the best of my understanding, claims to promote prevention, but the type of work and recommendations that it provides are related to something different. Information from this board's own website indicates that since 1948, it has had a few name changes and additions to what general areas it includes. Some of the terms included under this board are aviation medicine, occupational medicine (1955), aerospace medicine (1963), general preventive medicine (1983), medical toxicology (1992), public health, undersea medicine, and undersea and hyperbaric medicine (1999).[27] I do not intend to step on the toes of the individuals who work in any area of that current board. The board describes itself as "medicine specialists [with] core competencies in biostatistics, epidemiology, environmental and occupational medicine, planning and evaluation of health services, management of health care organizations, research into causes of disease and injury in population groups, and the practice of prevention in clinical medicine. They apply knowledge and skills gained from the medical, social, economic, and behavioral sciences."[28]

I have read the paper from the National Institute of Health titled "NIH Consensus Development Conference Statement on Preventing Alzheimer's Disease and Cognitive Decline."[29] Representatives of preventive medicine were present at this conference, and the conclusions from the conference were dismal: "Currently, firm conclusions cannot be drawn about the association of any modifiable risk factor with cognitive decline or Alzheimer's disease." Realize that at the highest organized levels of science and health, you will not receive any hint or answer of what you should do to prevent the disease that is waiting for you.

I look at such a consensus statement and understand that some of the invited members may have tried to inject some aspect of prevention into the conclusions, but as happens in most political decisions, their voices were silenced. Perhaps some members of the conference wanted to instruct you to get your *carotid arteries* checked, find out the size of your *left atrium*, get a monitor of your heart to be sure you do not have unknown—asymptomatic *atrial fibrillation*, or be complete and thorough in evaluation of a *hypercoagulable state* with fourteen vials of blood. Then again,—perhaps not. As of this writing, you do not have any American board that is recommending true prevention for you. So I suggest to you that you are reading the beginning of an entire new branch of medicine: Medical Prevention.

I am describing a new branch of medicine formed out of the current physiological abandonment by doctors of their patients. With effort a physician of medicine could again return to you—providing the medical decisions more often than the health care decisions. Some doctors are simply paralyzed by medical decisions that have no basis of absolute truth—and yet not much in the history of medicine is considered absolutely true. That is why the profession is known as the art of *medicine*. I considered if we would ever look back to current medicine and refer to it as the art of *health care*.

A meta-analysis is a medical research paper produced from combining statistical evidence from multiple sources. These papers are not studies and do not follow the rules of science. Rather, authors look at other studies and try to draw conclusions. One needs to be *very* careful when looking at the conclusions that come out of meta-analyses. Meta-analysis is useful for finding a pattern in treatment and disease and helping to determine what else should be studied in science or medicine. I believe it is difficult for one to sort out what the data represent when one has only the conclusion of a meta-analysis. I think publishers should print them in different print or in a different color so that everyone who reads them understands that the authors could have collected the data of studies that were improperly designed and are now reporting under the guise of true science. I find it sad that often meta-analysis data can be corrupted into the headlines that we read. Once published, suspicions can do the work of truth. In 2005 epidemiologist John Ioannidis stated, "In modern research, false findings may be the majority or even the vast majority of published research claims."[30]

A severe weakness of meta-analysis data is that the designers of the paper can pick and choose what studies to include into their review, thus installing a significant amount of bias into the conclusion. By selecting medical studies that support their conclusion and excluding any data that contradict it, the designers of a meta-analysis can easily come up with results to suit their needs. So be careful when you see that information you are getting from your doctor or your national preventive task force is based upon meta-analysis data; they are controlling what they want you to hear by basing their conclusion on select medical studies.

Get an understanding of what "data" you are provided when you turn on the TV or pick up the newspaper. Here is a sample meta-analysis study that I designed to demonstrate how you need to be careful with data and facts as they are provided to you:

Look at Planet Fitness. It has a stepper section. In the stepper section there is a plain old box. You step up onto the box and back down to the floor for exercise. And here is my study:

"I took data from people who have used the stepper and others who have observed the stepper and its use. I compiled data such as height and weight, speed of use, and injuries that take place. I collected data about the ages of the people using the stepper. Participants filled out a medical questionnaire. Some participants received a small fee to cooperate with the study. A specific pattern developed that I wanted to look into. When I evaluated the confidence intervals, I determined that the data were *significant*. (This is a line often inserted into meta-analysis studies to try to build confidence that the authors are telling you something useful. Using the confidence intervals is a way that meta-analyses are able to gather statistical power.) Those who used the stepper were frequently overweight. I was able to conclude that using the stepper at Planet Fitness could make you overweight. "

And so I publish this data with the conclusions that I have drawn. Most people will get to look only at the conclusion or the summary and not at the data or how they were obtained. The logic and thought process behind many of the headlines you read are not so different from this example. A group will easily take some point it wants to prove and then go out and find the data and studies completed by other individuals, in the end taking that data and molding them into whatever results the group desires. In 2012 the FDA published new safety label changes for statins.[31] The document they authored contains many references to meta-analysis work and their conclusions integrate such data. Their work does not evaluate an individual product, rather it lumps all products into one pile. The FDA did not perform a new medical study of the subject simply a review of the literature. Based upon their references—In my own opinion—they made premature statements of an entire area of medicine that has not been properly investigated.[v]

Be careful when you see the word *meta-analysis*. This is not science. This is not medicine. This is prescience. This is premedicine. Keep it there! Use it if you like, but please do not draw any conclusions from what you have found in your results. You can use this to decide what you would like to study. Use the data to observe results that give strange patterns or strange connections. Then go out and set up a study for what you believe to be the conclusion. Do not base your conclusions on data collected for different reasons. There are too many variables. Just think of what it would do to a fitness club if a headline claimed "Using the Stepper Might Make You Overweight." Even if the headline says "might" and the article acknowledges limitations of the study and that some of the authors don't agree with the result, in the end crappy science could destroy a business. This is what meta-analysis can do.

The headlines reporting the "rising cost of health care" are not accurate. The increase in Medicare payments is not going to doctors. If you split payments into five parts (doctors, hospitals, insurance companies, Medicare advantage plans, and other), you see that much of the money is going to the insurance companies. In the end, many Medicare plans are elaborate and creative schemes to gather more money into the coffers of insurance companies. Often Medicare pays more for an individual's XXXXX advantage plan than it would if that individual

---

v   When an official organization simply mentions the name of a drug and a side effect in a document (even with words like *potential—generally—non-serious—reversible*) the action is enough to send everyone running up into the hills.

maintained a traditional Medicare plan. The same plan that gets a solid chunk of cash from Uncle Sam reimburses medical providers less than the accepted Medicare rates. Yes, this happens daily. Third-party insurance carriers have many ways to get the money from the government and not release it to the health care teams that provide the services.

If you are reading this and work for Medicare, please do what you can to prevent any further "subcontract" work from being done. Man up. Keep doing what you have been doing since 1967. Despite any type of administrative overhead, you are still the best show in town. Yes, as I write about Medicare, I do so as a doctor who is in one of the lowest Medicare pay zones in my state. I also write this as one who receives some reimbursements from Medicare advantage plans at a rate that is lower than the state welfare Medicaid program rates. Someone really dropped the ball there, giving all of the control to third-party insurance carriers.

"Evidence-based medicine" sounds like a really good concept, but if something has not been studied, the results from "evidence-based" scientific papers might be confusing. Often the conclusion of evidence-based research is "because no research has ever been done on this subject, we cannot recommend doing x, y, or z." Treatment pathways are decided by evaluating algorithms and using meta-analysis data. Often the USPSTF covers an entire area of medicine, specifically preventive medicine, in a way that sounds like proper homework was completed. But all they truly say is that no one has looked at this subject yet, and research is needed before anything can be concluded.[32]

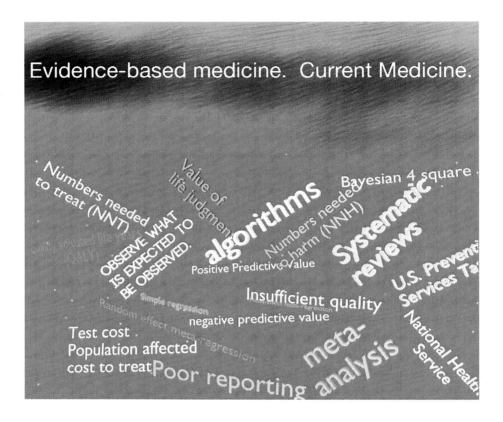

Others have published medical articles that speak of corruption in medicine. *The Lancet* (Vol. 359, no. 9313; 2002) is one example. The editors of this most-esteemed scientific journal asked, "Just how tainted has medicine become [by pharmaceutical industry payoffs]?" They concluded, "Heavily and damagingly so," urging "doctors who support this culture for the best of intentions" to "have the courage to oppose practices that bring the whole of medicine into disrepute." This is a component of the current problem, but pales in comparison to the rationing of your care by a for-profit industry.

6

UNDERSTANDING MY TERMS

This chapter could feel a bit random to you as you work through it, but realize that I am trying to acquaint you with my thought process. Once you understand where I'm coming from, then the rest of the book and chapters will sound logical to you. This is where I "throw down the gauntlet." I want you to understand exactly what you have never thought of before. Yes, this is a new way of thinking in medicine, and not everyone will agree with it. I will be explaining both medical terms and terms that come from my own opinion. I would be unable to convey my concepts to you without going into details for you; if you need to get back to your World of Warcraft game, then skip to the chapter on Alzheimer's disease and dementia.

I expect that when one speaks of prevention for someone else, nothing is done. Yet when one speaks of it for how one cares for one's own body, that person wants to prevent future pain and suffering.

Practitioners of *internal medicine, general medicine, family medicine*, and other fields all come out of the branch of medicine that is heavily influenced by guidelines; however, one cannot get good medical advice when looking *only* at guidelines. (Remember, guidelines are designed for the herd and not the unique individual.) When is the doctor going to be able to be the doctor again?

Cancer gives no warning. Most cancers are detected once they are in an advanced state. You will not have many signs or symptoms of a cancer that is working inside you until it is advanced, and perhaps even spread. Detecting the cancer at a time before it spreads is significantly better than detecting it once it has spread.

Most people's understanding of Alzheimer's disease is incorrect. People understand there is a term that uses the word *Alzheimer's*, which describes a memory problem related to dementia. But using the term *Alzheimer's* to describe memory problems in general is incorrect.

When people go to their doctors, they should hear the truth of their medical conditions to the best that the doctor truly understands or has looked into.

"Hey, I was at the doc's yesterday and he said that my heart sounded really good. Yeah, they did some blood work and said that I'm fine, nothing to worry about. —ohh— my cholesterol was a bit high, but nothing to worry about for my age they said. Yep, I got a good checkup."

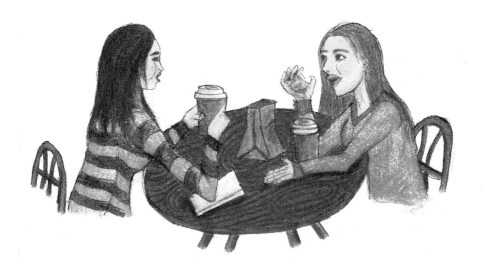

I would like to understand what this means. Without some objective data from accurate good-old testing (EKG; echo; carotid ultrasound; ultrasounds of thyroid, pancreas, liver, and kidneys; and something on the chart that reflects what is happening inside the stomach), well, honestly your doctor has no idea what is happening with you. Your doctor can only state, based on a brief and superficial examination, that you do not have any *evidence* of metastatic cancer. When a female goes to a physician with the pain of metastatic cancer, she receives a diagnosis of cancer. When one goes because of the symptoms of a metastatic cancer, one receives a diagnosis. When one goes to the doctor with symptoms of a cancer that has grown so large it is noticeable in some bodily function, he or she receives a diagnosis. But when a person hears that everything is fine, he or she really has no idea whether or not everything is fine. Not many cancers are detectable until they are already in an advanced state. But over a decade of discovering and treating a variety of cancers before they reach that state has proven to me how important it is to look beyond superficial evidence. Doctors who ignore the advantages of modern technology when working to prevent metastatic cancers are providing more health care and less medical care. Remember, you are unique. No one simple test covers all of the difficult prevention you need.

Many cancers can be detected while in the precancerous state.

Many cancers can be detected before they spread.

Once a cancer spreads, the treatment options become more difficult.

The cure is possible; **prevention is difficult**.

Most basically, a person has sixty organs that can develop cancer, and there are more than two hundred types of cancer known to afflict humans.

Many things in the world are tested and refined, and then they run like a machine. Often changes are made in an initial design to make the final product much better, safer, or more usable. Some parts of this book are designed to be put to the test. What you are reading is a work in progress and your appreciation of that will help you succeed in Medical Prevention. You need to expect changes in your approach as new technology is developed. What you do this decade for prevention may not be the same in the next.

While completing original academic research as part of this book, I encountered many difficulties. Academic research is expensive (investigation review board fees, participant fees, etc.). Designing a purely objective data study is difficult. I deeply appreciate the aspects of patient confidentiality and patient participation in a study. I believe, however, that so much effort to protect everyone's personal information is generally road blocking in research. At what point does an X-ray of a patient's hand no longer require the patient's permission to be used (without identifying data attached)? After the person dies?

One hundred years after death? It would seem that the bones of the Egyptian mummies don't even belong to them anymore; they have been moved across the world at the whims of others. When medical information doesn't include a direct name or identification, there is no reason it shouldn't be used for medical studies—disease tracking, patterns, and other uses. I doubt we will ever see the day that laws and regulations aren't constantly adding layers and layers to how academic studies must be executed. When so many details are required for moving forward, the wheels of progress grind to a halt.

The least expensive test is the one that makes the diagnosis. If you want to protest this statement, please be sure you have reviewed this work completely. If you are concerned about the corporate bottom line, then I cannot help you. This statement might be surprising, but you'll understand why I make this claim after you've read the work completely.

Medical reports should no longer use terms such as "within normal limits." (An early physician reviewer of this work commented that the abbreviation for this phrase—WNL—should stand for "we never looked.")

When a radiology team wants to help a doctor interpret a patient's data, it needs to describe what it sees in detail. Often a patient's current health care team does not want any detailed reports because it will always find other issues to deal with. Many health care teams are happy with a one-line conclusion, keeping their interaction with patients simple. When many diseases are not well understood, patients deserve more accurate and detailed reports.

By contrast, reflect briefly that for a report to become **MEDICAL PREVENTION CENTER CERTIFIED**, words such as *within normal limits* (WNL) or *age appropriate* cannot appear on the report. When radiologists read images, they must describe what they see. When pathologists read the histological slides, they must provide an explanation of what they see. Pathologists are not allowed to say WNL. Radiologists are paid to do a job. Radiologists who read reports for the **MPC** will provide substantive details, or they will not be reading your report. Some radiologists enjoy providing the proper details to allow a study to become **MPC CERTIFIED**, others see it as a burden.

Your health system is run by companies and industries that profit from rationing your health care.

I am not trying to fix the entire system, which serves its expressed purposes. I do want to fix the broken parts for you. If you love your mother or father and want to know how close they are to their first *micron stroke*, ministroke, or massive stroke, then follow what I explain. I do not want you to have a stroke either, so be sure to apply what you learn to all those around you. Preventing the first stroke is simple, but you need to do it. A monkey can make a diagnosis after your mother has had a stroke. The health care system has let you down.

"Stay out of the hospital; the hospital will hurt you. When you are done being hurt by the hospital, come and see me and we can figure out what needs to be done next. If you have a medical condition that requires a hospital visit, get in, get treatment for that, and get out."

This statement is my daily conversation with my patients. When my mother reviewed this book, she hated the idea of telling everyone what I say on a daily basis.

"Allen, you are going to make a lot of people mad at you."

Once a hospital administrator told me she tells her mother the same thing. My mother relaxed a bit after hearing that. The hospital does not intend to harm you, but in the process of providing 99.9 percent accurate care, mistakes are still made. Hospitals complete an internal study of medical errors and design ways to prevent those errors as best as possible. Changes and advances in technology will put the observation of medical errors behind the ability to prevent them.

It's impossible to grasp all the things that are working against you when you're in the hospital.[33] The nurses and doctors may care, but the hospital does not necessarily care about you or your medical needs. The hospital only cares that you do not stay longer than what is profitable for them. The term is *diagnosis-related group* (DRG). The administration of the hospital directs your care while you are in the hospital bed. The administration of the hospital needs to look at keeping the doors open while facing declining reimbursements from insurance companies, government-sponsored plans, and the ever-increasing uninsured. The doctors who provide medical care often have their hands tied by the hospital. Terms such as DRG, length of stay, intensity of care, level of care, readmission rates, and x-diagnosis codes do not mean anything to you if you are in need of medical care. All of your care in the hospital is rooted in the economic treatment of your disease or disorder. This economic treatment of your condition obscures any unique aspect of what makes you an individual.

That said, not every hospital admission is bad or wrong. Many good hospitals help people all day long, and I concede to them that they are doing a great job. For years, when I did my rounds in various hospitals, I was impressed over and over with how nursing and ancillary staffs were able to really *care* for the patients. I know if you are work for a hospital that you often wish you could do more for the people who are admitted. But political and economic factors, not scientific and physiological ones, work to water down care. A slightly different way of looking at this is to understand that when and if you are hurt by a hospital admission, do not be surprised. Medicine is not perfect, and often people expect that it should be. Many people believe they are checking into a five-star resort, rather than understanding the real details of what awaits them. The hospital is not exactly a war zone, but once admitted you should proceed with caution.

**"Concentrated power has always been the enemy of liberty."
—Ronald Reagan**

It was a sad time when health insurance companies trumped science in dictating how we care for people. Even during a time of economic turmoil, health insurance companies are still posting record profits. In the northeast United States, I certainly don't see any buildings left vacant because a health insurance company went under.

Most people are not interested in prevention. They do not want a change. They enjoy and like going to the doctors and being told they are fine. They enjoy hiding in the crowd and playing the odds. "Hell, it's only a one in ten thousand chance that it could be me." This is easy. This is simple. This is free. To many this is satisfying.

Prevention goes against the grain of health care thinking. Getting you to think of your body organs will often start to make you uncomfortable. People do not like to believe that anything could be wrong with their body. Many people feel pressure or anxiety as they consider their internal organs, knowing they have been ignored. Knowing how horrible some cancers end up being, many feel a sense of dread when they are simply considering their own prevention. On the other side of this coin is the excellent sleep you get when you realize that you do not have pancreatic cancer or stomach cancer. You might be up to the task. However, many of you will not be able to go down the path of prevention because of deeper psychological factors such as ego and pride. Some have a difficult time admitting they could have been ignoring a problem. You get to pick. I will make it an open door for you. Just step through the door. Enjoy what prevention can offer you.

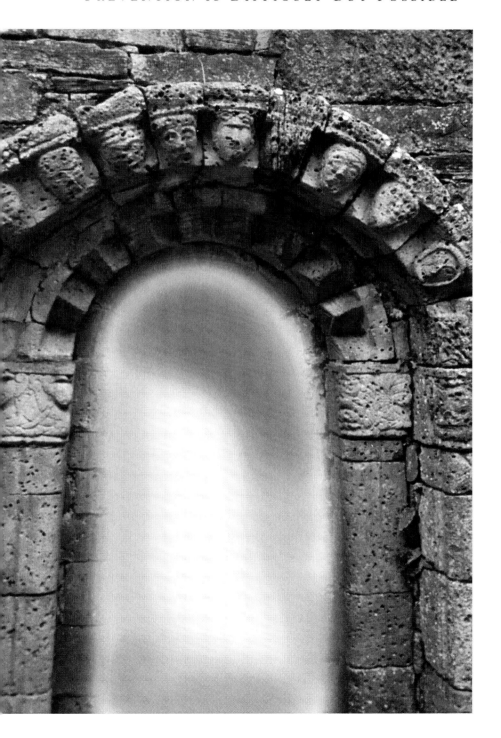

Testing/study/research results based on mortality are misguided. We will all eventually die. Concentrate on quality, admissions, and functional capacity. Look here. This is your human experience. Don't fret about the day of your death. Do not use the end as the goal for all you do. Enjoy your time here, and work with your body to secure good quality years ahead.

I will be critical of certain organizations, colleges, clubs, and task forces when they are lax. I intend no direct insult to you if you are a member of one of these academic facilities. I do understand that as a recommendation is passed, you might have been the one who voted no or who wished to state the conclusion differently. As you read this, you will appreciate being able to treat an individual as a unique person and give that individual a proper plan. Your health team should have based your original recommendation on prevention, not the financial bottom line. Remember, the least expensive test is the one that makes the diagnosis.

You need to understand that dying is not easy. I know that is a difficult sentence to understand, but many people will suffer a great deal before their bodies give out. Sometimes sudden death strikes a person, and it can often be a tragedy, but more often death comes after a great deal of pain and suffering.

At times writers of medical research papers do not gather the information to draw conclusions properly. Many factors influence medical research, and often conclusions are based upon incomplete data. Consider this example of why details need to be thorough: You have a red wall that you want to paint white. You apply one coat of white paint, and when you finish the first coat, you don't step back and say, "It's impossible to paint a red wall white." You certainly *could* conclude that. But you could also conclude that it takes more than one coat of white paint to cover a red wall.

When medical research papers are completed, errors in the conclusions are frequent. Details are often confused and inaccurate because of the large number of components that needs to be carried into the conclusion. If a medical research paper recommends treating people for their high cholesterol, for example, but doesn't recommend treating to an LDL of 50–70, then the writers of the research paper cannot draw an accurate conclusion.

In this work when I use the term *doctor*, you can simply interchange any of the following with that term: *health care provider, physician assistant, nurse practitioner, health care team,* or *provider*. Yet the term *physician of medicine* will often be used to explain those doctors who are not health care-supplying robots you have become used to. A subtle point, but there is a difference between a physician of medicine and a provider of health care—your personal experience will define your understanding as it relates to this point.

For this work you should know a few details about taking care of the plumbing inside your body. If you dump bacon fat down the kitchen sink drain day after day, before long you have a plugged-up kitchen sink. Your body's plumbing is similar. LDL is the bad cholesterol.

LDL above 130: you get a disease from poor plumbing (dementia, heart disease).

LDL between 100 and 130: you still get disease of the carotids, along with dementia and heart disease—but at a rate slower than if your LDL were above 130. And you will need to not have any other risk factors (diabetes, hypertension).

LDL between 70 and 100: you likely won't have any plumbing-related diseases. (Remember that additional risk factors can still give you more blockages.)

LDL lower than 70: if you have eliminated other significant risks, the blockages in your body will dissolve. (Yes, you can make that 20 percent carotid artery stenosis go away by proper and detailed medical treatment.) If your LDL is lower than 70 because of your lifestyle alone, then I love you—you are rare and take good care of yourself!

The data that support this LDL evaluation are provided in a separate work that is underway, indicating a decade of dedication to studying LDL and the disease states that are caused by it. I will leave this as my personal experience over time for this medical situation for this work. Once the data and conclusions are peer reviewed, I will look for publication in a journal.

Many people make lots of money from these diseases. Continue to read this book; it will affect trillions of dollars. This money could be spent on infrastructure and improvement of the United States. It's mind-boggling to think of how much money is spent on health care worldwide.

If the data are true—and the cost over years is trillions of dollars in the United States alone for a variety of disease—that is a lot of money. If we spent less on health care, we could spend more on other things. And isn't that what we're looking for—economic activity and recovery, a way to become the greatest country in the world again?

Many statistics have been formulated to calculate how often a disease affects Americans. Example, there almost two hundred thousand silent first myocardial infarctions each year (a heart attack that the patients don't know they even had!). Every twenty-five seconds an American will have a coronary event, and every minute someone will die from one. Almost eight hundred thousand people will have a new or recurrent stroke every year. Data from 2006 indicated that strokes caused one of every eighteen deaths in the United States.

Detecting a cancer in an otherwise well individual will always be better than not detecting it or ignoring it until it becomes noticeable. Yes, some will try to explain away the presence of cancer, suggesting that the affected person may have died from some other unrelated disease state. At times this does happen. But you should be careful when making such generalized statements. Whether a person dies from cancer or something unrelated, testing for cancer is still a good idea. And often what appears to be unrelated isn't (a pulmonary embolism, for example, is often tied to cancer).

Say you are one of those doctors or health care providers who has CAT scan, MRI, or ultrasound in your own "house." Well, I might say "shame on you" a bit. I might also say "good deal." Usually, I believe you are ordering many tests that the patient doesn't need. If you, as the medical provider, recommend a test because of financial incentives—shame on you. I would expect that the doctors you hired to read those tests are also part of the same group and benefit every time you order a test. There should be rules that prevent this from happening. A health care provider should have "arms' distance" when looking at the financial incentive built into ancillary service care.

This work is generated out of frustration with the lax guidelines that task force recommendations produce. The plans that they have set into motion all but eliminate the common sense of simple patient choice. Gone is any science or physiology of medicine from the treatment plans. Insurance companies performed a coup d'état on the medical community, and prior authorizations and formulary use are the proof. Windfall profits to these same insurance companies should spark everyone to open their eyes about the politics that dictate their medical care. I send this work to you with hope it will generate a good conversation with your doctor and health care team. You will also be able to decide if you are getting medical care—or health care.

59

When I speak of "others," I am referring to anyone or any group that does not have the same perspective as I do. "Others" could be task forces, specialty colleges, insurance companies, government agencies, or local policies. I am not trying to imply that "it's my way or the highway," but simply that "others" have made their mark in the sand, and I plan to call them out on it.

Body organs change according to all that they are subjected to over the years. Some organs show the result of continued insults from the environment and our own behavior. Skin on the arms of an older person affected by years of sun exposure is usually thinner and can bruise easily. But you will not find this same problem on this person's back, which is generally protected from the sun. So you cannot blame skin degradation on age alone. You can speak of how an organ responds to a specific insult over time, but time itself does not directly impact many of your body tissues.

I sympathize with many radiologists who want to perform quality work and whose detailed reports would raise a number of unforeseen questions. When a radiology team reports findings with unknown causes, the health care team might criticize the radiologist and perhaps demand a deeper explanation and a rereading of the report. The health care system allows no room for a radiologist to report, "We are just not sure, but you should do a good evaluation for any known causes of this finding. If you do not discover any known cause, then consider monitoring this condition and following it over time." A radiologist's pay should be based on the details provided in the report, not on whether that radiologist can explain every detail.

I believe that many will be more comfortable evaluating their own prevention needs privately. Speaking with someone else about your needs and limitations is difficult. Deep in the human psychology, one finds more difficulty admitting that something could be wrong in front of others; however, alone you may be able to consider these things more peacefully and less defensively. None of us wants to admit to another that we have not been taking care of ourselves properly. Our egos want to believe that what we are doing is best. We want to believe that how we are taking care of our body is flawless. We want to trust that our health care team is giving us only the most perfect, personalized advice. It's difficult to admit that there may be a better way and that the advice we're getting may not be exactly correct or proper.

Once you realize that something has been overlooked, you might feel uncomfortable. It's true that no one is a "know-it-all," but when an ultrasound of the ovaries is not even done, you can end up a "know-nothing." If you do not look, you will not know.

Just about every contractor has to get an idea of the work that a subcontractor does. Someone who works in construction will know after a few years which contractors he can trust and rely upon and which ones will give him trouble. It is the same in medicine. When you want accurate results of a test, then you need to have a good understanding of who is doing the test.

When I was in my residency, I hated journal club because of how dry the other people were when they presented their data. When you read things you have an interest in, you can consume them. When the data given to you is on a subject you care little about, then it can be torture. If the subject is of little interest to you, then you will really have no understanding of whether you are provided the truth. What was so bizarre is that once I was in private practice, all I wanted to do was read journals. I think it occurred after I realized that the news didn't necessarily reflect the truth—or even common sense. A few articles really sparked me off and then I realized, "Hmm ... what data can I trust? Well, if I don't read it, don't see it, don't see the facts, don't get to read the facts, how the study was designed, how it was written ... then the conclusions are blocked till I get that far."

Some studies are written specifically to reach a specific conclusion and not to supply data. For this work I have included some landmark studies that were completed, but I will show you how simple faults in the data can significantly change the results. Even as I write this work, I cannot believe that multibillion-dollar companies have such little understanding of the work that they do. Luckily for me, the studies they released are in solid black-and-white print, and I can show you simply where the errors are, and you can decide on your own.

7

PAIN AND SUFFERING EQUATION FOR COST

When one adds in the pain and suffering of some of these disease states, the "savings" of preventing the diseases becomes tremendous. Pain and suffering are never included in the cost of providing you your health care when "they" refer to your health care as a resource. In a civil lawsuit, however, the law considers pain and suffering to be valid injuries that demand compensation. I question whether any of the American academies have ever been in litigation for which their recommendations, when followed as a guideline, specifically missed disease states that were easily detectable. I wonder if the physicians who took care of patients who developed disease states that were easily preventable by simple tests had any recourse in referring to guidelines. Likely not.

I believe that when it comes to solving problems in the worlds of computer software, electronics, engineering, and various other industries, many would agree that the least expensive test is the one that makes the diagnosis. Spotting a problem early, when there is still time to do something about it, pays for itself. This is also true for you and your health. Yet financial considerations drive most patient care. In many industries and fields of business, costs/savings analysis is perfectly appropriate. But it should never be applied to people. For one thing, money is only one part of what something costs. As it stands in medicine today, the basic premise behind a decision to screen or not to screen is defective—it doesn't include pain and suffering.

In civil lawsuits and court rulings, pain and suffering, emotional stress, and inconvenience are valid considerations worthy of sizable compensation. But in medicine that is not the case. In fact, a review of nearly all the medical literature written in English fails to yield anything like what I am about to describe.

Side A (your current health care team): the cost of testing measured against how much it would cost to treat the problem.

Side B (MPC): the least expensive test is the one that makes the diagnosis.

One must consider the pain and suffering of the patient and family members. How much does it cost to visit your spouse, mother, father, or child suffering from a preventable disease in a hospital? How can you quantify watching a loved one waste away till bones show? How can you put a price on observing a loved one drift from pain into slumber, back into pain again? The patient receives painkillers to take the edge off, but rarely do they bring comfort and alertness at the same time. How would you rate the trauma of throwing up and not being able to eat because of chemotherapy or radiation treatments?[vi] Where is the price tag on the lost spirituality, compassion, creativity, and empathy?

---

vi   Not attempting to support letting cancer spread, but over the last years, patients I have cared for tolerated chemotherapy and radiation therapy very well. Cheers to the advances in agents used and techniques.

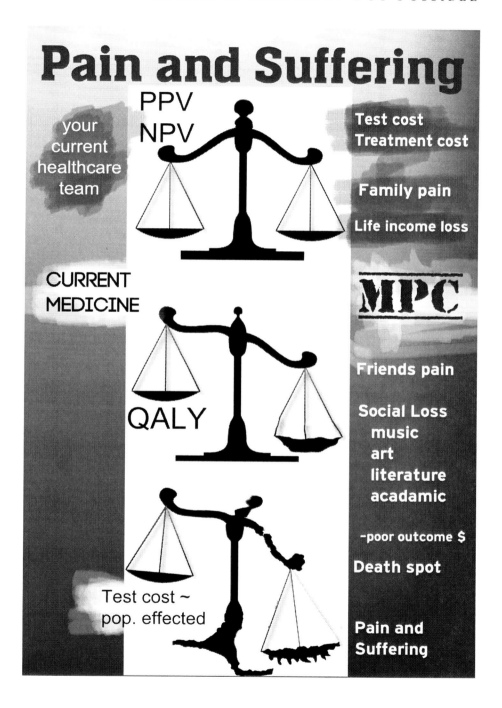

Often people are directly involved with the tragedy that is the pain and suffering of a metastatic cancer. After speaking with people, I hear a common theme: "So my grandma had pancreatic cancer, and she died a horrible death from it. I guess I was lucky that I was in Spain at the time, but my sisters keep telling me how good it was I did not have to see her like that. In a way I think it was good I missed all that rough time."

So I ask a question of the individual: "Well what have you done to make sure that you don't have pancreatic cancer? What has your father done to make sure that he doesn't have pancreatic cancer?"

The same answer comes back to me: "Oh, well, he goes and gets checked out for all that stuff, and I'm sure that if there was something, then they would find it. You know he is always getting to the doctor and taking care of things."

That is the exact conversation that many of you could have with me.

In 2010 the financial cost of stroke and cardiovascular disease in the United States alone was estimated at $503.2 billion.[34] When you add in the cost of pain and suffering to those billions, the savings of preventing these diseases are immeasurable. Once pain and suffering are considered, the cost of having a disease far outweighs the cost of testing for it.

Several factors go into creating screening guidelines for different disease states. On Side A is the cost of testing to detect a condition before it is bad, balanced against how much it will cost to treat the problem. Some of the factors that go into the decision are positive and negative predictive values (PPV and NPV), quality-adjusted life-years (QALY), test costs, population affected, and the cost to treat the affected person. A group sits down to evaluate the money that is spent or saved. Members of the group evaluate the cost of providing a screening test and the effect on a population living longer. Some better evaluations also include the quality of life. Often the data that the group uses to synthesize its final plan are faulted, as the data were not specifically designed to study the question the group was asking. Often a medical study is completed with one set of goals, and then another group takes that data and attempts to integrate it into its guidelines.

(If you have no interest in understanding statistics, then skip to the start of the next chapter. The rest of this one may feel like a boring class. Really, I warned you!)

When dealing with statistics, a term called the *positive predictive value* (PPV) is often integrated into the thought process behind ordering tests. The PPV is complicated when you apply it to a unique clinical situation with factors that you can't reproduce exactly every time. Most medical papers that use PPV to justify their specific intervention or guideline often do not address the entire issue. Often an author can end a conversation with showing how PPV data support the conclusions. I will not be providing you much PPV data. If you want medical treatment combined with statistics, then you can seek many other completed works.

You also have the option of deciding whether you want your health care team to provide you information based upon quality-adjusted life-years (QALY). Your health care team should clearly explain your treatment decisions based upon QALY, as any tradeoff needs your expressed consent. Even current recommendations for dealing with breast cancer are based upon cost.[35] When you meet with your health care team, be sure to understand whether the advice you receive is unique to your situation or whether you have been squeezed into an equation designed for a mass of people. Statements such as "Odds ratios and 95 percent confidence intervals, adjustments for age, then stratified by major ethnic groups" reflect some of the thoughts that go into Side A of the equation. I have a difficult time trying to understand how some of those factors can help you.

When a doctor uses end points of mortality in designing a screening process, it can confuse things even more. We should be considering quality of life. The "number needed to treat" (NNT) equation is one a doctor uses to evaluate the effectiveness of a health care intervention. This is epidemiological information. I believe that the appropriate place for an NNT calculation is in the use of a drug. When one considers a person treated over time with a specific test, then an NNT calculation can assist. Any type of screening test has calculations of sensitivity and specificity.

Negative predictive value and positive predictive value will also be based off a Bayesian 4 square. The Bayesian 4 square is made up of the numbers of true positive, false positive, false negative, and true negative results. The square is the usual tool that is used for statistical evaluation of data. I realize that once someone starts to speak of statistical information, most people just switch off. I am sure that the calculations all have a place to be used. However, I also believe that they can complicate certain disease states—by trying to make them simple enough to fit into a four-by-four square! In applying the statistical evaluation to a screening test, there is no easy way to calculate the power that a proper treatment would provide over time. In reflecting on the NNT equation, one can then include the lasting benefit of long-term treatment.

Side B: The illustration shows many aspects of what needs to be considered in any type of prevention medicine, namely pain and suffering of the patient and patient's family. The true cost of this component is difficult to measure. Kings would hand over entire kingdoms to avoid some medical conditions. What good is all the money in the world if you cannot use it? We should consider the cost of treating any problems a test may reveal. Often treating a problem in an early stage will cost much less than treating it once it is advanced. An example of this is finding a tumor and removing it surgically while it is a single nidus, as opposed to performing surgery, giving radiation treatments, and administering chemotherapy for a cancer that has spread through the blood and lymph systems.

We should also consider the likely results of a given test. At times the medical system errs and subsequent prevention measures harm the patient. The potential for this often scares people into thinking that finding a medical condition leads to unneeded procedures. True, if your health care team does not know how to interpret data and apply proper follow-up, you could be hurt. But conscientious and thoughtful evaluation of test results does not lead to unneeded procedures.

At times the loss of a person to a preventable disease inflicts a cost on society. This includes the loss of music, art, literature, science, and academic works the person could have created had she survived. An early death from a preventable problem weighs on society even more. The location of the death can become emotionally charged. People avoid the spot on the soccer field or basketball court where a young athlete died suddenly. Consider this the death spot. The stigma associated with these locations can last for years.

Some medical conditions are not preventable. Current technology has limitations. The potential for human error—misinterpreting data, for example—makes treatment even less exact and certain. It is unclear how to deal with this, other than making sure that each person involved in a health care team is provided enough incentive to do her job the right way.

This work does not give you a financial plan for saving your life. This book is about you and what you can do. I am not telling you a country will adopt a policy of preventing dementia and then save trillions over the next ten years. But it would be nice if it did.

8

ASYMPTOMATIC DISEASE

I would love for everyone who reads this book to find some direct connection with the content of this chapter. It is important that everyone understand that not everything has a warning sign.

If you went to your auto shop, and your car was returned to you with only five of the six lugs on the wheel, I am sure the guy at the shop would say, "You're fine." But you would look at that and say, "What the hell?" So why do you accept "You're fine" when your doctor does no evaluation and only meets the expectations of insurance companies? Your doctor in this example is a good provider of health care—but no longer a physician of medicine.

Anyone reading this work no doubt has access to a computer, which performs a boot test every time you turn it on. Your computer is able to go through a complex diagnostic testing of many of the aspects of its little life. But when you get up in the morning, you don't get any error messages. You don't get a warning and then an option to hit F1 to continue. If you did, then perhaps you would have a good idea when a problem is starting. But usually you don't get any messages from your body until it is already too late. You body is designed like that, to ignore pain.

Asymptomatic is a tough term. We need to delete a few terms from the medical community because of improper use. *Asymptomatic* tops the list of overused terms. When a doctor simply does not detect a disease because the health team has paid no attention to it, one should not call that disease asymptomatic. The termites in your basement are asymptomatic, but once you find them, you have a big problem. The tick that has bored into the skin of your back, but you do not feel, is asymptomatic. Diabetes is mostly asymptomatic, yet we treat it. Hypertension is mostly asymptomatic, yet we treat it. When asymptomatic refers to a known disease state that a doctor closely monitors, then the term is valid.

A good example of something that is asymptomatic is an indolent lymphoma. (This disease can have a long clinical course; early treatment and delayed treatment show about the same results, so actually for this disease, waiting for symptoms is not as harmful as for other diseases.) In this situation asymptomatic is appropriate because the disease is known and has both an expected clinical and symptomatic history and a well-understood treatment plan.

In the medical community, often inappropriately, professionals use *asymptomatic* to explain a disease that currently afflicts a patient but without symptoms. No one knows that the disease is there. But just because we do not look for a disease does not mean that the patient is asymptomatic. No one would consider waiting for high blood pressure or diabetes to cause symptoms before starting treatment, so why is that the procedure for so many other medical conditions? If you do not look for a problem, then the result is asymptomatic—that is, you don't have a problem.

For the most part, task forces are designed not to look for any diseases. Without looking for early stages of diseases, people will get those diseases. I doubt that members of task forces were ever on a house call for a patient dying from metastatic breast cancer. I have been there. A simple mammogram in a woman at age eighty-two would have detected a precancer—and cutting the lump out could have cured her. (I can hear the wheels turning and the mental grumbling of some of you who think that eighty-two is old. You may be thinking, "Man, why is this guy treating people who are that old? Just let them be; give up on them already." Well, if that is your mindset, then this work is not of much use to you.)

Asymptomatic means the disease is there but has been not noticed because no one has looked at it yet. When do we ever do this in life? When do we ever just not look and assume there isn't a problem. Your computer boots up and warns you of even small problems. The dash on your car tells you when there is a slight problem. Every aircraft has full monitoring of every component and fluid level. Every day in your life you make an observation and verify your results. You would not wait for your cell phone's battery to die before charging it. Well, if your cell phone were a patient in today's medical care it would not be hooked to a charger till it went blank and dead. You deserve better, which is why you are reading this work.

We spend our lives monitoring things around us without waiting for a problem. We monitor them to take care of problems before they develop. We call this prevention. This is difficult. We spend a great deal of money every day on preventing things from happening that we don't want to happen. We wear shoes to prevent foot problems (a $2billion-per-year industry). We wear hats to prevent a cold head. We wear seatbelts to prevent injury in the case of a crash. We lock our doors to prevent theft. We check the expiration date on milk to prevent drinking sour milk. Quite simply, we prevent hundreds of things hundreds of times a day without ever thinking about it. We spend time, money, energy, and thought on prevention for all sorts of things around us, yet we spend very little time on preventing diseases in our own bodies. Put me to the test—for a month, do not check the expiration on the container of milk! You can't do it (if you drink milk).

Your carotid arteries need attention. You should know exactly what is going on in there. How big are those blockages? How have they changed from the years before? Are they gone yet? Did you successfully dissolve those blockages? The part of the book where I explain this data to you will shake the medical literature world. I have dissolved carotid artery blockages many times.[vii]

I am coming from a different world of thought when I tell you that prevention is possible but difficult. You will have to do a lot of work and spend a lot of time. Most of your work will be in gathering information on the contours of your internal organs and linings of the alimentary tract. (Ultrasounds, scopes, and MRIs can be your friends). Those who embark on the task of dementia prevention will have an additional list of work that includes MRI, neuropsychiatric testing with interpretation, and other detailed homework assignments.

Preventive medicine in the United States is at best a joke or a laugh. The ways that insurance companies try to pay for performance move money around but don't help people much. The most troublesome diseases of the past—stroke, heart attack, Alzheimer's, breast cancer, lung cancer, and diabetes—still rank extremely high despite a number of years of pay for performance reviews and incentives. Current preventive approaches

---

vii   There was nothing simple or quick about it—often it takes years and a motivated patient.

are said to fail because they do not integrate the proper aspect of asymptomatic guidelines into the philosophy.

Even guidelines by the National Cholesterol Education Program Adult Treatment Panel (such as the NCEP ATP III) fall short.[36] When you attempt to identify different risks of disease without looking and checking for that disease, you simply miss the chance to prevent and cure. NCEP has been operating since 1988, and decades later the world is still plagued by high cholesterol. I do appreciate the most current recommendation for getting LDL lower than 70, but the NCEP needs to do better work of identifying people for whom this is important. The Adult Treatment Panel III (ATP III) of the National Cholesterol Education Program has been giving recommendations over decades. A detailed review of one of its recent guidelines generates some excellent prevention medicine questions. When the authors created their plan, why did they not include a specific way to determine high risk? To determine who is at high risk, doctors need detailed information on the condition of the carotid artery. One should understand who already has blockages. The authors do mention atherosclerotic disease; however, they list it as "clinical." I imagine that they wait for it to be symptomatic.

To present a strong recommendation and guideline, they should study the effect of leaving LDL above 130 over time. I am confident that all of the diseases that one would want to prevent would appear over time when you leave your LDL above 130. Sadly, many will also get these horrid diseases even with LDL 100–129 because of additional factors.[37] [38]

I appreciate that by twisting data in an epidemiological study and crossing with a study that was not specifically designed for this purpose, researchers could come up with whatever conclusions they desired. The Heart Protection Study (HPS) and PROVE IT were not designed to specifically study what the ATP III gave guidelines on. My point here is simple: researchers should study a subject and draw conclusions from what they studied. They should not reinterpret data from a different study and include it in an unrelated guideline. ATP III authors should have used the data from the five major clinical trials included in their guideline and then should have made decisions on what subject matter they would have liked to investigate. With the reference section including more one thousand references, I am sure the budget for a project like this spared no expense. Finally, one may wonder if results from their guideline will be published.

When one is going to launch into a study of an asymptomatic disease, the time invested needs to be more significant than generally expected. If the study is only two to three years long, the researchers could miss the expected results. My experience and data related to the medical dissolving of carotid artery stenosis cover a decade. Such valuable data allow us to understand that small changes on an annual basis have an additive effect over time. One can take a 20 percent carotid artery stenosis and completely dissolve the blockage, but it might take six years. What were you going to be doing anyway over those six years? You might as well dissolve the blockage in your neck rather than getting the disease it will cause.

The biggest problem with the ATP III guidelines[39] is that they work with the understanding of treating "*symptomatic* carotid artery stenosis." They treat diabetes mellitus as a risk not waiting for symptoms. Everyone knows to treat hypertension before symptoms develop. Why doesn't ATP consider waiting for diabetes to be symptomatic to consider it as a risk? When doctors wait for carotid artery stenosis to become symptomatic, so much damage has already been done that it is difficult to prevent dementia. Clearly, if nationally funded organizations want to remain consistent, then they should not wait for a disease so drastic to become symptomatic before treating it.

Consider the electrical system in your heart. An electrical node in one of the upper chambers communicates with another node that is a bit deeper in the heart. These nodes communicate through the muscle of the heart with another set of wires. (Detail: The sinoatrial node is close to the right atrium, and the atrioventricular node is closer to the right-sided heart valve. The His-Purkinje system has the fibers that carry the electric signal to the heart muscle.)

To understand the electric component of your heart, consider this analogy: Your house has a main circuit breaker through which electricity enters from the power company and out of which extends wires that go to different parts of the house. The sinoatrial node of your heart is like the transformer outside your house, which admits electricity inside. The atrioventricular node is like the circuit breaker/fuse box. And the His-Purkinje fibers are like the wires that convey the electric current throughout the heart muscle. (Entire textbooks are dedicated to this electrical communication, and it is complicated. I am giving you a brief look only.)

Often people ignore the electrical system of their body for years or even decades even though we can evaluate the electrical system of the heart simply by an EKG and an overnight Holter monitor. These two inexpensive and simple tests—which have no side effects—provide you with significant information about your heart. When properly interpreted, ventricular tachycardia, atrial fibrillation, a simple abnormal run of premature beats, or other irregular heart rhythms could indicate a condition you were unaware of. Currently, most doctors would consider this finding asymptomatic, meaning that the abnormal beats of your heart are nothing to worry about. Many boards of medicine would criticize me and offer lengthy sermons about not looking for disease when it causes no symptoms.

I appreciate that philosophy, but I'm coming from one that wants you to understand the working of your body. Medical Prevention is about offering or using science to understand asymptomatic problems you have before they give you symptoms. Once picked up we can then evaluate it. These electrical heartbeats often indicate underlying medical problems of the coronary arteries or the heart valves. At times there is no significant disease of the heart, and the unusual rhythm is simply just the way you are at this time in your life. Check again in a few years and keep an eye on it. You probably want a simple answer to the question what does my irregular heartbeat mean?, but so many factors need to be considered. Some factors that I consider are the status of electrolytes, the size of the left atrium, blockages of the coronaries, number of years on protective medications, condition of the heart valves, estimated pressures in the heart, prior understood and identified medical conditions, thickness of the walls of the heart, and many other details that are unique to each person.

Asymptomatic carotid artery stenosis does not exist. Please feel free to read my hypothesis on dementia (page 113) and understand right from this point that any and all blockages in the neck are leading to problems for you. The people with these blockages are simply waiting in line for their Alzheimer's disease, dementia, or stroke. Often an MRI of the brain will show white matter changes. Even in current times, most doctors do not appreciate what white matter changes are.[40] Modern radiologists, as a group, simply relate this finding they do not understand to the "aging process." But white matter changes are not related to age. They result from damage to the brain over time. High cholesterol (LDL above 70) and carotid artery stenosis change the brain and kill off cells. (Other factors also increase these white matter changes.)

Most of the time when I ask someone, "So how is the condition of your carotid arteries?" they say that they are fine, yet they have never looked. They simply rely on the superficial treatment that their health care team provided them. The computer that is your brain is dynamic, and even hundreds of ministrokes can go undetected by you and your doctor. Without looking for evidence, it often takes a full stroke or aggregate brain damage to get your attention.

People trying to take care of themselves have to get past the roadblock of "I'm fine." You might believe you're fine, but unless someone looks for them, no one will detect the early stages of many conditions; they are considered asymptomatic. And even though you go to a doctor, get blood work done, and get tested, you might feel a false sense of security in your health. Realistically, unless you inspect your body thoroughly and give it the time and attention required for prevention, you are missing those conditions. You can understand much of your body through noninvasive testing. Have you ever had an ultrasound of your carotid arteries, with the results explained to you in detail? Did you get the velocities and a stenosis percentage? Or did your health care team tell you that everything is fine? Worst case is that someone told you, "There is no evidence of any hemodynamically significant carotid artery stenosis." The poor, ill-fated souls who received the last bit of data are doomed.

Without careful testing and interpretation—like we do at the **MEDICAL PREVENTION CENTER**—your health is relatively unknown. You need high-quality vascular testing and a physician who specializes in or follows the philosophy of this work to interpret the results. Some day doctors will again be trained properly, and you will be able to get excellent advice by looking at the initials after the name. Currently, you might be stuck with a doctor who loves the term *asymptomatic* because it means that the health care team has to do absolutely nothing for you: "On to the next patient, we are done here."

Someone who believes in prevention understands that terms such as *no evidence of hemodynamically significant, within normal limits, asymptomatic,* and *not significant* often indicate false results. Some member of your health care team needs to read the test line by line and verify its accuracy and report the results properly: naming the percent of blockages in your neck. Most vascular tests yield "no hemodynamically significant carotid artery stenosis." You need to change those words to what they really mean: "We do not have to cut the neck of this person yet; he has more time to build bigger blockages before we start a plan." Doctors who understand even basic blood-flow physics appreciate that it is impossible to calculate what they consider not hemodynamically significant because there are two carotid arteries providing flow to the brain!

Consider how many young adults die suddenly during a sports event. There is no single registry that keeps track of how many children die each year from sudden cardiac arrest, but estimates are from one hundred to one thousand.[41] "Up to half the time in such cases, there are no warning signs in a child," said Victoria Vetter, MD, FAAP, FACC, of the Children's Hospital of Philadelphia. "The sudden cardiac arrest can often be the first symptom." Sadly, she went on to state that more studies are needed.

Wes Leonard died after scoring the winning basket in March of 2011 in Holland, Michigan. The past is full of many of these tragedies. What strikes me about this case was it happened just hours after I was speaking to a colleague and trying to make a point for a proper evaluation of youth who want to participate in sports. No national guidelines exist. Often a pediatric medical office will not even have an EKG machine.

Another way to understand the concept of asymptomatic is the Leaning Tower of Pisa. It is asymptomatic until it falls over. Once it falls over, it has symptoms. But even though at present it is only asymptomatic, the Italian government spends millions to keep it from getting worse. Your heart disease remains asymptomatic until it becomes symptomatic—which may mean death or disability.

New transient ischemic attack (TIA) guidelines are found in the AHA/ASA: 2009 publication.[42] One will again find that only "symptomatic ischemia without infarct" is considered. Because the medical custom is to begin work only when symptoms arise,

your current medical care is missing most of the damage being done to your brain. But you will not notice the damage being done because it is asymptomatic. Stroke will finally be prevented when one starts to look for the disease where it can
be found. My book emphasizes the importance of what I call
micron strokes. If modern medicine continues to ignore *micron
strokes*, then you should not expect any progress in the prevention of dementia. You can quote me on that.

When I modify medical advice based upon the age of patients
and what they have done in the past for Medical Prevention, I
have not yet been wrong when it comes to identification of an
asymptomatic disease. It is impossible to be completely healthy
from head to toe for your entire life. As time passes, the trillions
of cells in your body adjust, and you need to know when something is going wrong. If you happen to have no detected medical or physiologic problems at this time, I ask you to fast forward
a few years and repeat your evaluation. Whatever problems
you will develop as an older person are silently underway right
now.

9

PSYCHOLOGICAL ABANDONMENT

Psychological abandonment is a term used throughout this work. Currently, the level of psychological abandonment of patients by their doctors is so pervasive that the population has widely accepted it.

Published guidelines can be wrong and therefore harmful. Data suggest that pulmonary guidelines published in 2011 for pneumonia increased mortality. If verified, this means that the guidelines were both wrong and caused harm.[43] When one is able to identify that a current published guideline is wrong and harmful, one must wonder how many other guidelines are hurting people. How does your health care team use guidelines?

Patients across the world will cheer when no insurance company is able to dictate to doctors any aspect of the care that they provide. Psychological abandonment occurs when a physician takes care of a patient but does not really take care of the patient. The doctor is there, but she is not there. The doctor treats the patient but not to the best of her ability. Currently in the United States, this is an addictive epidemic. Doctors who work for health care companies are forced to make medical decisions to better the bottom line of the corporate books and not to make decisions that are the right thing for their patients. Many doctors even receive financial penalty to their pay or salary if they do not do exactly as their boss wants. Similarly, if a doctor does exactly what the health insurance company wants, the doctor receives a bonus. This means, and I am sure you have heard of this before, that a doctor cannot always use a specialist that she feels is needed, cannot write for a drug that the patient might benefit from, and cannot order a test or lab evaluation that the patient might need. I am not going to apologize if you are the unique health care provider who is working "for the man" yet able to give the proper advice to your patients. You, my friend, are rare and you know it! (Besides, you totally understand and agree with what I just wrote.)

In this work I explain to you how the United States Preventive Services Task Force takes no active role in preventing disease that you could currently have in your body, but rather, it puts you into a statistical pile of other people. You are a dollar sign at the bottom of the list. I know that my words on these pages may seem harsh, but I would be more than happy to sit down with anyone who writes a guideline that ignores common sense in favor of saving money. Often advice to patients is even worse. At times recommendations are based upon data and reports that are not designed to draw such conclusions! Shame on the authors for publishing such drama. Shame on the authors for publishing recommendations that will end up causing patient harm.

Other authors, such as Ruth Purtilo, have written on this subject in detail.[44] One cannot be sure there is any simple solution. Enjoy further detailed reading on this important subject as you wish.

I would love to spend pages and pages going on about contaminated vaccines,[45] [46] [viii] but the vaccine process has a critical role in prevention. I fear that in trying to explain some of the horrid things that have happened over the years, you would then interpret that all vaccines are to be bunched into the same suspicious light. Mandatory vaccine programs are, for the most part, just wrong; everyone should have a choice of the level of risk they want to live with. Yet not immunizing a child for an easily preventable disease is also terrible. The future will tell us what mistakes were made and what choices were the right ones. To be candid, I have little faith in any mandatory vaccine program. Whatever happened to patient choice? Mass immunizations are always risky. The gist is, simply think carefully about what you are doing, and don't rely upon a recommendation from an academy. We will be sure to disagree later in the book if you are of the mindset that getting a partially tested flu vaccine every year should be mandatory. (Yes, they get some degree of testing regulated by the FDA, but it is far less than what I would require for something that is injected into the body). We know little of prions and various biologically active particles transmitted in vaccines.[ix] Thousands of these particles have not even been identified, so proceed with caution when you get a vaccine.

A vaccine that prevents a few days of missed work should carry a different weight from a vaccine that prevents a more significant disease. A vaccine that offers eradication of a disease should be considered differently from one that simply serves the magnanimous purpose of not getting those around you sick.[x] For some who need the reduced risk of flu, immunization is a benefit. But forcing entire populations is not likely a productive idea.[47] Keep in mind some of the failures of mass immunization programs in world history. What happened when we massively

---

viii   Google search of "contaminated vaccines" yielded about 3,250,000 results (0.15 seconds) on 12-8-2011.

ix   Vaccine nanofiltration ~20–50 nm.

x   On its website, the CDC explains that it doesn't even know how many people die from the flu each year.

immunized Africa for polio? What happened when years later we massively immunized Africa for smallpox (using shared bifurcated needles)?[48] Forty million bifurcated needles were used to give out 2.4 billion doses of smallpox vaccine. Events can occur that are not the intention of the vaccination.

Because this is so controversial of an area, this is about all that I would want to say on this subject! Now I have to go get my tetanus shot.

10

ALZHEIMER'S AND STROKE

**"If the brain were so simple we could understand it,
we would be so simple we couldn't."
—Lyall Watson**

Most will understand and know how to identify a stroke (CVA). Less understood is silent cerebral ischemia (SCI). Many will be able to explain what is commonly described as a ministroke, a transient ischemic attack (TIA). But when I ask what is smaller than a ministroke (damage to brain, no symptoms, nothing visible on imaging), even experienced health care providers return with no medical term. Micron Stroke is the term I suggest. The micron stroke is an event that can happen without your knowing. There is currently no way to test for or image a single *micron stroke*. As your brain is damaged over years by more and more *micron strokes*—the effects become visible on MRI. A term called *silent cerebral ischemia* generally refers to findings on brain imaging that we can see. We cannot see *micron strokes* as a single event.

Some doctors and researchers initially retort at this new term as, "He is talking about something that we have known for a decade." Proceed with caution from here, as often the same researchers, after grasping all of the potential new areas that can be researched, start to understand the value of the term where there was not one before. Supplying a new concept in medicine is similar to cleaning up honey with a dry paper towel—it takes a long time and it is not easy. Doctors love what they can see and test for—an X-ray that shows an abnormality—a lab test showing an abnormal value—This is solid information easily understood. Evaluating a concept that they cannot see or test for leaves most moving on to other projects. I know there are many brilliant research people in the world, and they can arrange a way to test this concept, to evaluate for either single *micron stroke* or for the effect of thousands of *micron strokes*.[xi] I know animal lovers may hate the idea—But this is what lab rats are designed for—new concepts that have the chance to change how we understand medicine.

There are new concepts in this chapter that may initially be difficult for you to understand, not because they are complicated, only because they are different from what you already believe. If I were to write this chapter to cover every question that comes from this discussion, then this book would have another hundred thousand words to cover all the angles. New concepts need to grow in their own way. Simply, I need you to understand that there is a different way

---

xi   I suggest using multiple eight to twenty micron-sized particles of cholesterol plaques in an animal model. Observation of the histopathologic changes over time could open the door for additional understanding of how the brain responds to these insults. Brain MRI should not be able to detect the insults, yet histology will show the evidence. Additional studies can include the other causes of micron strokes. You, I, and a few workdays—we can set this all up.

to look at some of the things that you are already familiar with.

In 2010 total worldwide cost of dementia was estimated at $604 billion. "If dementia care were a country, it would be the world's eighteenth largest economy, ranking between Turkey and Indonesia. If it were a company, it would be the world's largest company, exceeding Wal-Mart and Exxon Mobile."[49]

What is more likely? A disease that we can't figure out or a disease that has a known cause that we are simply ignoring?

Most dementia is caused by factors—which we can group into nine primary categories—that cause *micron strokes* to the brain. —Allen J. Orehek, MD, **DEMENTIA PREVENTION CENTER**

MICRON STROKE HYPOTHESIS:

Evaluate brain tissue
Atrial fibrillation
Hypercoaguable state
LDL
Carotid artery stenosis
Tobacco
Hypertension
Diabetes mellitus
Systemic inflammation

Secondary Categories

Over time the *micron strokes* add up to form significant disease. In addition to the nine primary categories, I have identified dozens of secondary factors that contribute to dementia. Most of the *micron strokes* go unnoticed by the individual. The *micron strokes* show up on MRI as white matter changes once they number in the hundreds or thousands. As more and more white matter changes occur over decades, larger plaques form. Unlike the rest of the body, the brain does not have access to collagen and fibroblasts to form a scar. The histopathology findings consistent with Alzheimer's disease are similar and related, and perhaps even the same finding as found in other types of dementia. Most white matter changes are insidious— you will have no symptoms. Often you do not even know this process is occurring. Over time, as additional insults are provided to the brain, mostly without your having any symptoms, dementia starts. Dementia and white matter changes go hand in hand.

MICRON STROKE DEFINED: A single insult to the brain parenchyma by any etiology that cannot be detected either clinically or by an MRI. (Example: a single micron stroke of 22-micron size will not be detected). A cumulative effect of multiple micron strokes, when they number in the hundreds or thousands, is detectable by MRI as white matter changes and atrophy. Conglomeration of micron strokes ultimately can be detected as white matter changes. Micron strokes the size of a capillary (8 microns) up to smaller arterioles (30 microns) could occur at the rate of hundreds or thousands before conventional imaging or neuropsychiatric testing detects them.

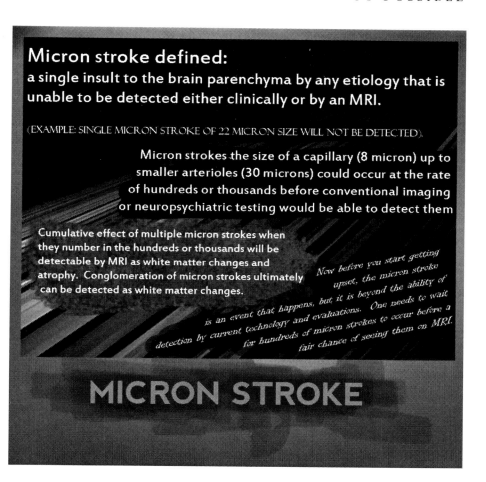

Micron stroke defined:
a single insult to the brain parenchyma by any etiology that is unable to be detected either clinically or by an MRI.

(EXAMPLE: SINGLE MICRON STROKE OF 22 MICRON SIZE WILL NOT BE DETECTED).

Micron strokes the size of a capillary (8 micron) up to smaller arterioles (30 microns) could occur at the rate of hundreds or thousands before conventional imaging or neuropsychiatric testing would be able to detect them

Cumulative effect of multiple micron strokes when they number in the hundreds or thousands will be detectable by MRI as white matter changes and atrophy. Conglomeration of micron strokes ultimately can be detected as white matter changes.

Now before you start getting upset, the micron stroke is an event that happens, but it is beyond the ability of detection by current technology and evaluations. One needs to wait for hundreds of micron strokes to occur before a fair chance of seeing them on MRI.

MICRON STROKE

I deny that the brain has to rot as part of the aging process. I have authored a paper that directly challenges theories of any "aging process" of the brain. I am sure that if you do not take care of the brain, you will develop the "aging process" that is often referred to and openly accepted as unavoidable. Our brain is not well understood; many scientific and physiological mysteries surround it. I believe that damage to the brain can happen over time, but there are no set cellular changes that occur with time. As they come out of the bone marrow, the red blood cells of a seven-year-old and an eighty-four-year-old are hardly different. There is no rotting or aging process that happens with red blood cells—your red blood cells do not get older as you get older. One cannot look at the red blood cells of an eighty-year-old and say, "this is blood from an eighty-year-old"—So why is medical literature full of "brain-age disease?" This point is so strong to me that the **DEMENTIA PREVENTION CENTER** is working on a scientific paper related to this topic.[xii]

While working and doing the research for this book, I wrote *The Micron Stroke Hypothesis of Alzheimer's Disease and Dementia*, published in *The Journal of Medical Hypothesis* Volume 78, Issue 5, 2012. (doi:10.1016/j.mehy.2012.01.020). With hope, this scientific paper will create an international discussion, perhaps leading to prevention or attenuation of this devastating problem of dementia. You can join the discussion at micronstroke.com.

Dementia is preventable.

Prevention is difficult—the cure is possible. Nine primary factors and dozens of secondary factors are well beyond the ability of your current health care team to respond to. You will not find a fancy simple guideline. Preventing dementia requires the skinned knuckles, sore feet, and dirt under your nails that accompany all hard work. As each case is unique, the number of hours involved in reviewing and integrating all of the data into your final risk is unknown. I know you want a quick answer here—sorry, it doesn't exist. You are unique!

HOLD ON TO YOUR LIFE: You are literally holding your life in your own hands. You are sliding down the rope through life, and when you reach the bottom of the rope, dementia occurs. Your rope can break or you can slide all the way to the bottom of the rope—you get dementia. The rope that you are sliding down has two aspects, length and thickness. Where are you holding onto that rope? How far have you slipped close to the bottom? The longer the rope the better; the length gives you some lee-

---

xii   Paper is related to the topic of looking at brain MRI images and being unable to detect the person's age with any accuracy, thus making a diagnosis of age related inaccurate. Paper is in study stage; some data obtained.

way to slip here and there before reaching the end of the rope. The thicker the rope, the better; you have a stronger rope to hold onto. The primary pathway determines the length of the rope.[xiii] The secondary pathway issues determine the thickness of the rope.[xiv]

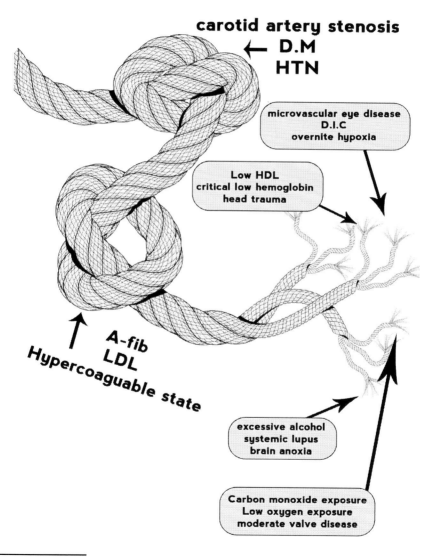

carotid artery stenosis
← D.M
HTN

microvascular eye disease
D.I.C
overnite hypoxia

Low HDL
critical low hemoglobin
head trauma

A-fib
LDL
Hypercoaguable state

excessive alcohol
systemic lupus
brain anoxia

Carbon monoxide exposure
Low oxygen exposure
moderate valve disease

---

xiii   Large knots: two are shown but your rope has at least nine.
xiv   Smaller strands of rope—dozens of strands, one for each possible factor.

You are holding on for your life as you know it. Consider the rope you want to hold onto—feel it in your hands. Place pressure on the rope as you allow some of your weight to be pulled down. Envision the length of the rope that you want to hold onto. The longer the rope, the better. This is your rope. Pick a good solid rope and hold onto it. If you need help setting up a thicker or longer rope, then work on what you read in this book—it will help you prevent your rope from breaking or reaching the end of the rope. Once you know the condition of the blockages in your carotid arteries—you will have evaluated at least one knot on your rope.

There are over one hundred years of medical information and details to integrate and explain. If you want a simple answer, it would serve you better to ask me how you move part of your body at will. I would generalize and explain that it involves signals in the brain, nerves, and muscle fibers—but that would be such an over simplification that no justice to what really happens would be given. To understand how to prevent dementia, you need to understand the basic parts of the process. Be prepared. Even explaining this on a basic level can be confusing. Here you go!

Alzheimer's disease is a type of brain disorder diagnosed with a brain biopsy. In modern language, Alzheimer's is a term used to describe memory problems. The term is commonly applied to people who have dementia. Understand that the word Alzheimer's is used as both a term and as a disease diagnosis. When Alzheimer's is used as a term to describe a type of dementia, it is not completely accurate. One needs to be accurate when it comes to the treatment and prevention of any disease, especially one affecting the mind. Dementia is a huge problem in the world today, and we should approach it with scrutiny. Not all of the dementia in the world is Alzheimer's disease. Many people have been misdiagnosed. Landmark studies that take decades to complete still fall short of helping us confirm causes of this problem.[50]

Outline of the phases behind the cause of dementia.

Phases of the process of dementia and treatment.

1) Understand what Alios Alzheimer described in 1906.

2) Understand that Alzheimer's is a disease and Alzheimer's is a term.

3) The disease of Alzheimer's may have no cure –

4) The term Alzheimer's when used to describe a type of dementia is preventable!

5) Alzheimer's is diagnosed by brain biopsy.

6) Even with brain tissue the pathologist can still be confused.

7) The histopathologic diagnosis has no "Gold Standard."

8) There are many causes of dementia.

9) Many causes of dementia are bundled incorrectly into Alzheimer's diagnosis (used as a term, as there was no brain biopsy completed)

10) Some of the dementia are mixed with Alzheimers's disease, as a guess.

11) Consider why the healthcare team used a guess as a diagnosis.

12) Feel frustration at why a "guess" was used for a diagnosis.

13) Get a bit mad and realize that your loved ones deserve better than a guess.

14) Open your eyes and realize that if the dementia awaiting you is different from Alzheimer's – then why you are not doing anything about it!?

15) Unless you make changes, your preventable and treatable cause of dementia will be misdiagnosed as an untreatable disease.

16) The dementia in your future can be prevented.

17) The dementia in your loved ones future can be prevented.

18) Hold on to your life.

19) Start the process of preventing dementia now.

20) Get started on preventing your dementia by exploring the specifics of what causes a Micron Stroke.

21) You have 9 primary categories, and dozens of secondary issues to deal with - take your time - be complete and pay attention to the details.

22) Your dementia prevention could be beyond the capacity of your health care team to deal with - you need to be motivated - you need to understand the disease process better than your health care team.

In 1906 Aloes Alzheimer described a disease in the brain of a fifty-five-year-old woman. The dementia process he identified is what we now commonly refer to as Alzheimer's disease. Over a hundred years later, we still make the pathological diagnosis in a similar way. (Those who named the disease after Alzheimer must have known what they were doing because even the name causes great confusion.)

Dr. Alzheimer studied extensively the process of the brain called atherosclerosis,[51] a specific disease state with neuritic plaques and neurofibrillary tangles.[xv] It is widely known that both neuritic plaques and neurofibrillary tangles are not unique to Alzheimer's disease.[52] A pathologist is a doctor who looks at tissue samples under the microscope to tell you what a diagnosis could be. In the world of the pathologist, there is no certainty about what one could call Alzheimer's disease and what one could relate to another process.[53] [54] [55] This small fact simply shakes all that we believe we understand about this disease.

As a term, Alzheimer's is applied to *almost all* people who lose their ability to think and remember short term. The term is often incorrectly applied. Very often we hear that there is no treatment of or prevention against this horrible problem.[56] I will stress to you again that this is not true. Remember that Alzheimer's is misdiagnosed more than it is properly diagnosed because no one is out there doing brain biopsies! (And even if they were, no one is sure what definitively classifies Alzheimer's.) Yes, dementia is real, it is horrible, and it is all over the place. But dementia has many causes, and Alzheimer's is only one type. Given that it requires a brain biopsy to make the diagnosis, many people receive this diagnosis as a *guess* from their health care team. The largest danger in this guesswork is that many health care teams overlook many types of treatable dementia.

Once a patient receives a diagnosis of Alzheimer's, the health care team goes into a watch-and-wait approach because there are no good treatments for Alzheimer's. I do not want you to be upset with your health care provider, but now that you understand Alzheimer's better, you know more than the doctor taking care of you and your loved one. I will say that again

---

xv   Such terms describe the findings when evaluating tissue with a microscope.

in a different way—now that you understand that Alzheimer's is a diagnosis that a doctor makes exclusively through a brain biopsy, you are correct in questioning the many Alzheimer's diagnoses you are probably aware of.

As there are many causes of dementia, your next step is to start eliminating the ones that your doctor is missing. Yes, this is going to be up to you. I hear you saying, "But they must know this, and I am sure they are looking for all types of dementia and aren't just guessing here, are they?" Guessing at a diagnosis that causes so much pain and suffering for everyone around? Guessing at a disease that costs trillions? Yes, the diagnosis was a guess, and in making such a guess all of the pressure is now off your health care team to provide anything useful because there is no cure. Do you see how simply that all fits together? When your health care team guesses you have an incurable disease, there is no work involved and no need to do anything further. As for you, you are different now—you are reading this work, and you understand that you will not just be pushed along like cattle.

Recently, the Alzheimer's Association and National Institute on Aging issued the first new guidelines in twenty-seven years to diagnose Alzheimer's.[57] Three expert international work groups no doubt spent a lot of time and effort preparing this work, which will probably open doors to additional funding and research, but they have not provided any useful clinical information for your health care team.[58] [59] [60] New plans by the Obama administration—drafted by the Department of Health and Human Services in 2012 may not have the impact you expect on the problem of dementia. Efforts appear to concentrate on medications, diagnosis, and financial/caregiver issues—but not prevention. Sad for many—but for you, prevention is here in this work.

In evaluating a variety of published information from the National Institutes of Health[61] on dementia, one will find that, as discussed earlier, many people do not receive the correct diagnosis of their type of dementia. Terms such as *vascular dementia* or *multi-infarct dementia* are closer to describing the millions who are affected. Either way, the dementia is the important part that you should concentrate on while you are completing and reading this book.

Some types of dementia are not treatable or curable, including cognitive dysfunction in multiple sclerosis, normal pressure hydrocephalus, Binswanger's disease, Pick's disease, frontal lobe degeneration, the dementia associated with motor neuron disease, HIV-related cognitive impairment, Korsakoff's syndrome, Huntington's disease, Creutzfeldt-Jakob disease, and progressive supranuclear palsy. But the most common cause of dementia is preventable. You can prevent this disease, and thus you have a cure. If it takes root, you can stave off the symptoms, preserve functionality, and perhaps even regain some brainpower. Prevention is of paramount importance for anyone who does not want to lose his or her mind.

Presently, the only way to definitively diagnose Alzheimer's dementia is with a brain biopsy. Not every case of diagnosed Alzheimer's dementia is the correct diagnosis. Recall that even at the time of the biopsy, not all pathologists will agree on what they look at would be considered Alzheimer's disease or another process. Many scientific journal articles have been written related to this subject. Many articles do not disprove my hypothesis that the smallest insults (**micron strokes**) to the brain from a variety of factors add up to larger plaques, neurofibrillary tangles, and senile plaques. [62]

Do not think of dementia as a specific diagnosis. You do not just get dementia one day. This problem is not like a rash that was not there last week but suddenly appears. It exists on a spectrum.

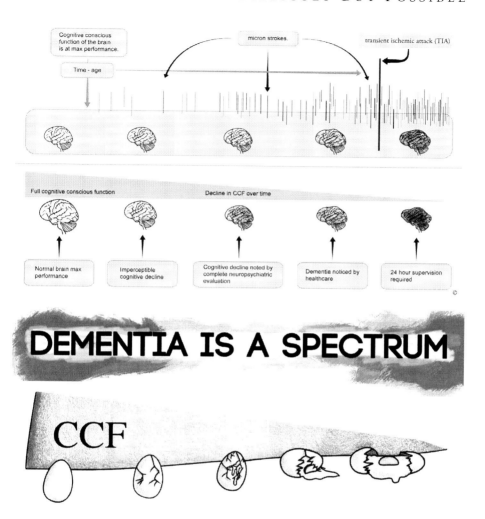

You start out someplace in life with your cognitive function, and as your brain suffers from *micron strokes*, you lose your cognitive ability. Waiting for your health care team to identify your cognitive conscious function decline leaves minimal time to mitigate this disease.

Stroke affects all age ranges but is found mostly in older people.[63] As the population of a country ages, more people are at risk. So what are you doing to prevent your first stroke? You can start with an ultrasound of your carotid arteries.[xvi] You can have your stomach checked out—with an EGD or similar test—and if there are no reasons that you cannot take a baby aspirin, then do it! Aspirin has a benefit that stems from its work as a platelet inhibitor. Once you know the condition of your stomach, you are then fully able to enjoy the baby ASA each day without being worried that you will be one who develops some type of gastric or stomach bleeding. You need a secured stomach. Then starting a baby aspirin could be right for you. Secure your carotids and treat that disease.

I have completed a literature review of English language medical studies using search criteria related to esophagoendoscopy, ASA/aspirin, and gastrointestinal bleeding ("What are the gastrointestinal bleeding risks and complications of taking ASA 81 mg p.o. [per os, by mouth] daily after one has had an EGD that evaluated and treated any existing conditions"), and nothing suggests that it has been studied. When you consider a daily dose of aspirin for prevention, you need to be sure you are starting with a stomach lining that does not have any diseases. If you do not verify the status of the stomach, you are simply taking the chance that "all is okay." You deserve better than taking a chance. Be sure that your stomach does not have disease before you enter into a long-term treatment plan. Diseases of the stomach include, ulcer, gastritis, helicobacter infection, polyps, Barrett's esophagus, esophagitis, GERD, and more.

The link between Alzheimer's and dementia and how to prevent is complicated. Nine primary factors and dozens of secondary factors are involved in the *Micron Stroke Hypothesis*.) The initial understanding has to come from the fact that there are two main arteries in the neck: the carotid arteries. These arteries supply the blood to the brain. After age forty, many people develop blockages of these arteries (some people

---

xvi   To be effective here, you need to have an ultrasound of the carotid arteries that is **MPC** Certified™

develop these blockages before age forty, but these are less common). The carotid arteries develop blockages as a result of the bad cholesterol in your body. This is referred to as your LDL. Your body makes this bad cholesterol in response to the foods that you eat. The blockages start out small. As time passes with an elevated LDL, the size of your blockages will increase.

Detecting the exact size of the blockages is simple yet highly technical. Testing needs to be done with a well-qualified vascular lab. Many locations and hospitals do this test but report suboptimal and incomplete reports. A number of grading systems are in place. The typical gradations are 0 percent (which is no blockage, no plaque), 1–19 percent, 20–40 percent, 40–80 percent, and anything above 80 percent. The majority of prevention takes place when blockages are below 20 percent. Once this disease is in the 20–40 percent range, you have already had many ministrokes. They will show up on your MRI of the brain as white matter changes.[64] An important point here is that the blockages in the lower ranges do not cause any blood flow abnormalities, so they will often be labeled "nonsignificant carotid artery stenosis." You really need to identify the abnormality of your carotid artery in the earliest stage possible. This abnormality is essentially a ticking time bomb. If you have these blockages, and most of you who are reading this book do, you need to get a set plan to treat and dissolve the blockages. Your regular health care team's plan is to wait for the blockages to develop into more significant blockages. Once you have developed significant blockages, then you will be given chances for treatment.[xvii] But you will have missed your chances to avoid the damage to your brain.

One of the difficult facts for current medical literature to grasp is that blockages of 1–19 percent have already started to do their damage to the brain. Most patients with blockages in the 20–40 percent will have already had white matter changes and

---

xvii   Treatment can be a carotid endarterectomy, surgical removal of the plaque from the neck artery.

ministrokes, and all blockages more significant than that are guaranteed to have had ministrokes. The patient may not feel or notice these *micron* and ministrokes, but over time they add up. An MRI of the brain confirms the damage of blocked carotids: white matter changes. Scientific evidence supports this.[65][66]

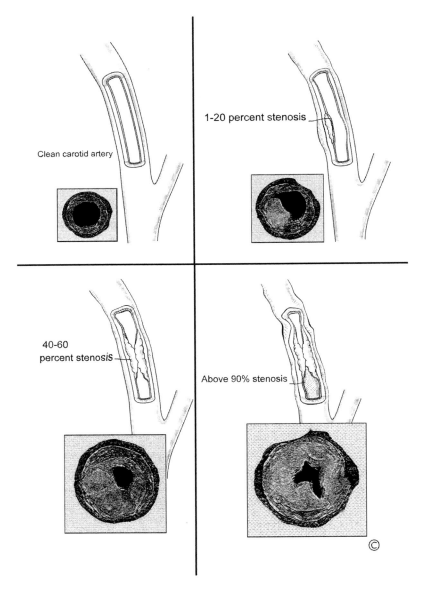

Clean carotid artery

1-20 percent stenosis

40-60 percent stenosis

Above 90% stenosis

©

The next significant link is that the *micron strokes* and ministrokes over the years develop into what is commonly referred to in the United States as Alzheimer's disease, or dementia. I have already discussed with you that most of the Alzheimer's disease is improperly diagnosed because no brain biopsy was completed. To distinguish other forms of dementia from Alzheimer's, formal neuropsychological testing is a very good option. Detecting mild cognitive dysfunction during your testing is your start to preventing dementia. I do not suspect that your health care team will suggest you go for neuropsychological testing unless you push for it. A basic rule is to go for neuropsychological testing if you have white matter changes on your MRI and any of the other nine primary factors that lead to dementia.

I recommend rating *micron strokes* according to the size of the blood vessel that is involved. Capillaries are 5 to 10 microns in size. Therefore, a stroke in a capillary is a 10-micron stroke. A stroke in an arteriole would be a 20-micron stroke. A stroke in a larger artery would depend on the size of the artery, which could be from 100 to 5000 microns. Why are strokes classified in a general manner in current medical terminology? There is a significant difference between an 1800-micron size stroke and a 100-micron stroke. I believe that this fact has never been studied, but this makes good common sense. The effects of a 100-micron stroke can be more noticeable than that of an 1800-micron stroke, but that is just how the brain is. Some stroke locations are more powerful. Even the most complete physical examination can miss significant damage to some parts of the brain .

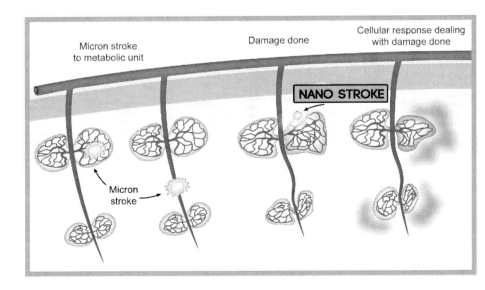

Diagnosis of what is commonly called a ministroke, or TIA, is complicated. Once there has been some improvement in a patient's initial symptoms, the water becomes muddy. Many ministrokes are explained away every day by health care teams because, once a patient has recovered, there is no way to determine what happened in the past (although an MRI of the brain will show a pattern of increasing white matter changes with more events).

Many medical studies have performed brain biopsy for evaluation of brain tissue after death. Often the medical studies find that the subjects had had multiple insults to the brain. Both physician and nonphysician parts of the health care team studied these subjects while they were alive.[67] One cannot assume that in all of these studies the health care contacts simply had no idea of how to identify an insult to the brain, so one must assume that insults to the brain often go unnoticed. With every paper I read, this point becomes more solid. I am sure that across the world it is the rare health care provider who can pick up the signs and symptoms of a resolved TIA.

Micron strokes and ministrokes are often undetected. A *micron stroke* or ministroke may cause a short period of numbness in the face or body. But please don't start freaking out because you slept on your arm and it's numb. That is not a stroke. Everyone can Google "stroke" and learn what they're like, and this book is not about helping the people with that problem. They have already missed their chance to treat it. But an episode of facial numbness could indicate a micron or ministroke.

Review of the current published medical literature fails to describe anything smaller than a TIA or stroke.[68] [69] [70] Those at the helm of stroke prevention, the American heart Association (AHA) and American Stroke Association (ASA), do not recognize *micron strokes* in their data.[71] [72] [73] [74] The American Academy of Neurology endorses the publications of the AHA/ASA. Those who are responsible for prevention of stroke do not fully understand and acknowledge all of the data. I am not implying that these authors' work is wrong, however. It is just imprecise. I am confident that there will be much agreement and many medical journal articles produced on this subject in the future. Some day you may find this term in medical guidelines, as authors of such scientific statements would love to be the solvers of big problems.

If you have no symptoms, then a TIA or a stroke will not be diagnosed. If you never get the diagnosis, then much damage will be done to your brain before symptoms (dementia) finally show up. My door is open to any of the authors of these publications who would like to refine definitions and expand what can be prevented.

New scientific studies should be performed that would assign a micron size to the stroke and then follow those affected over time. Both groups would develop dementia based upon the rate of their brain insults and the relative sizes of the blood vessels involved. I feel confident that with time the people with the more severe strokes will do worse and those with the smaller *micron strokes* will do better. I would call for better-funded centers to study strokes because currently anything smaller than a 600-micron stroke is all but impossible to clinically identify. I feel confident that someone brighter than I could come up with a grading system that is better than what we are currently using. A new grading system will include brain insults on the scale of 8 microns all the way up to 5000 microns. Even more exciting is that technology advances will continually improve our brain-imaging tools. If our fundamental thinking about disease states such as stroke does not start to change, then those afflicted will have a difficult time preventing them.

The excellent news for you is that should you go forward and be meticulous enough in preventing your dementia, you will prevent many other diseases along the way. If you are able to pick up on blockages in the carotids before too much damage is done, then you can dissolve the blockages with medical treatment. Once you have treated the blockage and dissolved it, you can monitor it from more of a "back burner" priority in your life. Until you get to the point of clean carotid arteries, I strongly recommend that you set your own goals rather than rely on any current medical guidelines. Sadly, not many health care guidelines will even review with you the condition of your carotid arteries.

We can identify and treat blockages with cholesterol-lowering medications and other options. For all but one in ten thousand individuals that I would see in my practice, I recommend a medication. My typical favorites are Lipitor/generic, Crestor, and, Zocor/generic.[xviii] Some new data from the FDA with Zocor does seem a bit weak to make sweeping recommendations.[xix] I have never noticed a significant bump in effectiveness from

---

xviii   I often add a product called Zetia once a patient is on his or her goal dose of a statin but LDL is still too high.

xix   Product was studied and used in a population open to drug-drug interactions. When interactions occurred, there was a label use change. Since 1992, some health care teams simply have restricted use in such drug-drug danger zones as they understood the pharmacology of the product they were using.

Zocor 40 to Zocor 80; no doubt, there is some improvement in LDL, but it is not an amazing change. Newest data from the FDA have confused/restricted the drug so much that it is unusable anymore because of so many contraindications.[xx] Welchol is an option to get the LDL lower in motivated people, and it is not a statin. FDA recommendations in 2012 need to be followed with proper medical studies. My personal opinion would add many chapters—as of this writing I do not agree with their March 2012 data release. You may agree or disagree with me—either way dementia will grow and affect you if you do not make changes.

When I have patients with an LDL above 130 and 1–20 percent carotid artery stenosis, they have a long way to go to their goal (LDL 50–70). I will usually look to a more potent product, along with heavier realistic lifestyle alterations. I don't think the other statin-type cholesterol medications are effective in this situation. If a health care team is able to get one of these products to work, reaching the LDL goal of 50–70, then fine, stick with it. But in my experience, only the products I named have ever brought a patient's LDL to between 50 and 70.[xxi] Still, if a patient prefers a different product, I am happy to try—when goals are set. If the patient is not able to dissolve the carotid artery blockages or if she is unable to reach the goal of 50–70 LDL, then we sit down and change course. (Remember, always get advice from your health care team. I am a doctor, but I am not *your* doctor.)

In looking at the men and women in the illustration, can you tell which have started on their way to Alzheimer's? Can you tell

---

xx   Cytochrome p. 450 is a large group of enzymes. Drugs that affect the physiologic pathways and interact with these enzymes will always need close observation. Zocor was approved in 1992 with use that could cause such drug-drug problems when health care teams prescribed them without knowing such interactions.

xxi   LDL goal of 50–70 is easily obtainable by a health care team across thousands of patients when approached by a method and thought process similar to mine. This LDL goal study has WIRB approval and is in early stages of planning. Completion by 2015 is my goal.

which of this group have already had *micron strokes*? Can you tell what their carotid artery blockage is like?

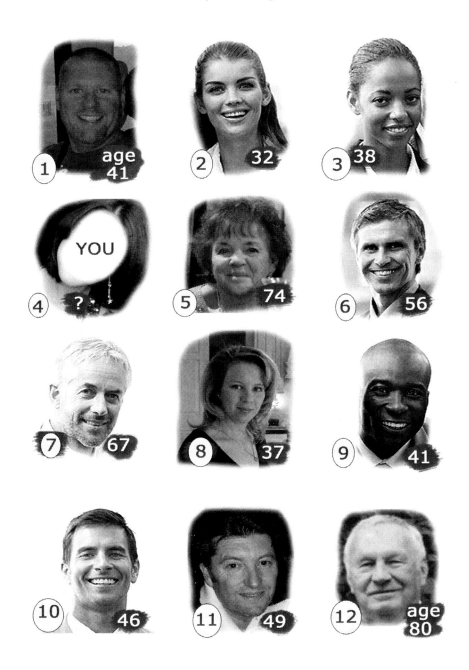

First, I want you to select from the twelve individuals those who do not have carotid artery stenosis. Take a moment and decide who does not have carotid artery stenosis. Next, realize there are only three without carotid artery stenosis in the illustration. Which three did you select?

The answers are 1, 5, and 8. Perhaps the question was a bit unfair, as you did not know the medical conditions related to each image. Number 2 was a diabetic since age seventeen. Number 3 started smoking when she was twenty-two years old. Number 5 is Rose, who has visited the **MEDICAL PREVENTION CENTER**. She started with 1–20 percent in 2004, and in 2010 she was back to zero. Typical results are in the range of five to seven years. During this time, an individual had ideal control of multiple health aspects, including no tobacco use, LDL 50–70, diabetes with HGA1C less than 6.5, and systolic blood pressure goal 119 mm Hg.. Number 6 and Number 7 never took any type of medication for their cholesterol. Both men lived their lives with LDL 120–140. Number 9 had systolic blood pressure between 130 mm Hg and 150 mm Hg since age twenty-nine. Number 10 started to use tobacco at age fourteen and quit at age thirty-six. Health care teams always told him that his cholesterol was a bit high with LDL 148 mm Hg, but without any other risk factors they never offered medical treatment, discovering that he had 90 percent blockage in the left carotid artery was a good day for Number 10.[xxii] Number 11 has 1–20 percent but is quickly working on getting back to zero. Number 12 enjoyed his tobacco use from age twenty till forty. He had coronary bypass surgery in 1976 and then a repeat coronary bypass surgery in 2004. He currently enjoys his life with 20–40 percent blockages on left and right.[xxiii]

I strongly recommend that if you are over age forty get to know the condition of your carotid arteries. And the only way you can

xxii   Number 10 was then able to fix his severe medical condition before taking a massive stroke. A surgery that cuts the neck and removes the plaque is often considered with such large blockages, carotid endarterectomy.
xxiii   Since 2004, LDL 40–60.

learn is by conducting a complete and thorough ultrasound. The **MPC** has specific criteria that indicate whether a report is complete or not. My exceptionally strong recommendation to you contradicts the advice of the USPSTF. The USPSTF (and other organizations) recommends against screening for asymptomatic carotid artery stenosis in the general adult population.[75] I hope that I get a day when I can sit with these people and go through the details that they have been missing. I know that a group such as this must consist of bright and intelligent people, so it confuses me as to how they can make national recommendations that are so obviously deficient. I know I digress from the subject matter, but a task force must understand that there is not a simple, quick solution. Medical conditions are complicated and unique. Currently, the task force is working with a box of Legos with forty parts; what they need to be working with is a box of Legos with four thousand parts.

Why am I so skeptical of guidelines? Perhaps it's because I have spent years obsessing over LDL levels and what it takes to lower them (specifically, lab data, patient education, and medications). I think it's also because as a younger physician, I often question the side effects attributed to medications, based on their specific physiology and how they work in the body. Sometimes the link is obvious, and at other times listed side effects do not add up. Regarding statin medications, I have never seen or identified a true allergy to these medications, yet the literature is full of "side effects and dangers." (I could write a whole chapter about what physicians should be doing to identify potential side effects while still having wicked success with such medications. I expect to include this in the LDL paper in progress). When grouped together, most data would no doubt suggest that there are side effects throughout the class. But when you consider the drugs individually, you will see that each has a different potential for side effects.

Patients with high cholesterol are given medication and told to exercise more and eat right. How many things are you planning on changing about a person without side effects? How many people have reported that they had a muscle reaction to one of these medications when really what happened is they had a muscle reaction to the exercise that they recently added into their lives? Leg cramps can be a side effect from medication—but leg cramps also happen when you exercise. The majority of these people are not getting the proper amount of exercise before they visit the doctor, and they start a new medication and a new exercise program at the same time. There are so many medical conditions that can be mistaken as side effects to a medication: exercise-related muscle fatigue, muscle growth and building, spinal stenosis, sciatica, peripheral vascular disease (blockages of arteries in the legs), back problems that send pain and cramps into the legs, arthritis of the knees or other joints, and a dozen other conditions.

I avoid this by starting with four to six weeks of "probation" time.[xxiv] When patients have extremely high LDL (above 160) or very high cholesterol (above 130), they are given the opportunity to do "everything for king and country" for four to six weeks. When they have new tests after this period, some of them are actually quite shocked and disappointed with mediocre reduction, and still some of them find that the LDL increased rather than decreased. But by allowing people this period to exercise, perhaps something they have never done before, they easily understand that any of the symptoms they feel in the legs and muscles are simply caused by their waking up and utilizing muscles. This is something that people expect as part of exercise: "no pain, no gain." Some people who are not much into exercising spend this time consulting a dietician. Even though most people do not like to hear that what they eat is bad for them, dietary changes are often necessary, but unrealistic. Most people will not change their diet very much. Most will continue to consume the same foods even though they are bad for them. So go see the dietician, and work through all that.

----

xxiv   Unless it is a new patient who comes to me after he or she has had a significant event, patients get statins on Day 1.

Sometimes, based upon initial results, I extend the initial six weeks to a full three months. After three months, the patient has adopted a new lifestyle. At times someone makes a quick sprint through six weeks of lifestyle changes and diet to try to get off the hook. Patients who do not reach their goals have a better understanding of their situation and are more willing to seek alternative ways of getting that LDL to lower than 70. A favorite quote of mine, and something I hope you take away from this book is, "Lowest dose necessary and shortest period of time." That is my calling card when it comes to the use of medications. People will go on medication but at the lowest dose. Then we recheck and adjust if necessary. As the years go by, sometimes people do make significant changes in diet.

Only one in ten thousand people who have more than 1-percent carotid artery stenosis will successfully lower their LDL to the 50–70 range through lifestyle changes alone. Usually these people are individuals who have rigid diets for one reason or another, which includes next to no refined sugar, enriched flour, or grain-fed meat.[xxv] When people are able to maintain a diet such as that, day in and day out, their LDL may actually reach a level that **MPC** and **DPC** love.

On national websites of Alzheimer's organizations,[76] the experts sometimes endorse early diagnosis. The benefit, as seen by these organizations, is that an early diagnosis allows the family to plan financially. I know that I am not the one who is breaking the news to you that the patient of patient's family will spend a lot of money. The bad news for those who make money from treating dementia is the fact that it is preventable.

---

xxv   Motivated premenopausal women under age 50 seem to have the most luck with lifestyle changes. Postmenopausal women who usually have carotid artery stenosis are not as lucky. A cruel trick of nature.

Micron Stroke Hypothesis of Alzheimer's Disease and Dementia.

Abstract.

Alzheimer's disease as currently described in the medical literature is often more a description of dementia rather than a specific disease. In over a century of scientific work there has been no proven theory as to the precise pathogenesis of Alzheimer's disease and dementia. As there is no efficient treatment for patients with Alzheimer's disease, prevention or attenuation of the disease is of substantial value.

An intricate collection of hypotheses, studies, research, and experience has made it complicated for one to completely understand this disease. The purpose of this hypothesis is to illustrate new concepts and work to link those concepts to the present understanding of an obscure disease. The search for a single unifying hypothesis on the etiology of Alzheimer's disease has been elusive. Many hypothesis associated with Alzheimer's disease have not survived their testing to become theory. Suggested here is that the elusive nature of etiology of dementia is not from one cause, but rather the causes are numerous.

Medical terminology used freely for decades is rarely evaluated in the light of a new hypothesis. At the foundation of this work is the suggestion of a new medical term: Micron Strokes. The Micron Stroke Hypothesis of Alzheimer's Disease and Dementia include primary and secondary factors. The primary factors can be briefly described as baseline brain tissue, atrial fibrillation, hypercoaguable state, LDL, carotid artery stenosis, tobacco exposure, diabetes, hypertension, and the presence of systemic inflammation. Dozens of secondary factors contribute to the development of dementia. Most dementia is caused by nine primary categories of factors as they interact to cause micron strokes to the brain.

Allen J. Orehek, M.D.

Many medical studies have been completed on the subject of dementia. Many studies try to cover too many facts and end up with poor conclusions. While preparing this work, I marked up studies line by line, pulled references, evaluated conclusions, and simply digested the data. If you are the author or investigator of one of these works, I intend you no harm. If my critique of your work needs further adjustment, or if you have facts that are not yet included, please let me know. This is a work in progress. Even the worst of the papers that I have reviewed still contribute in helpful ways. When Thomas Edison was asked about his failures in creating a battery, he responded, "I have not failed. I have found 10,000 ways that won't work."

A study[77] in 2002 on the "age-associated changes" in brain tissue claimed that the group of patients between ages fifty and eighty-nine had "no serious medical condition." Such a statement cannot possibly be true. The investigators did not evaluate all of the factors that contribute to dementia, so the results are faulty. I have identified dozens of factors that we need to evaluate before making such a statement. A more fitting statement would be, "Patients whose medical conditions are ignored develop brain damage as they age." I call for university centers and other funded locations to do their own study related to brain age and MRIs. I believe it would be truly astounding if an MRI of the brain would be able to tell you how old someone is with any accuracy. We could use the MRI of the brain to tell you how much damage someone has had to their brain. An MRI of the brain when completed and not thoroughly evaluated for the details misses the start of the dementia process. As radiologists read the MRI of the brain and rule out tumors and cancers, often they miss or improperly evaluate small vessel ischemic disease and white matter changes.

I have seen cholesterol collect in the back of the eye (very neat part of a physical exam when it is found). What data dispute that "deposits and tangles" might be the body's way of dealing with cholesterol in the brain?[xxvi] In the *Micron Stroke Hypothesis*, I suggest that further studies be planned to look for such information.

---

xxvi   Rhetorical question that requires research.

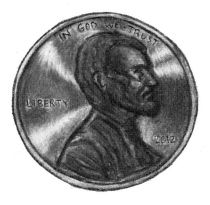
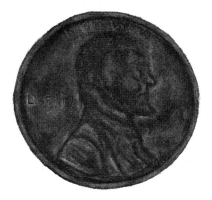

> Brains over time can be likened to the circulation of two coins. The coin on the left was across the map at trade shows and into a thousand hands. A simple coin protector allowed this coin into more hands than the coin on the right. The tarnished coin had no protection. Various degrees of use and abuse by the owners caused it to become scratched, worn, and damaged. Your brain is very similar when you consider the damage over time being done without protection.
>
> You do damage your brain over time, but your brain does not age.

I have reviewed CERAD Part I[78] and Part II.[79] I have read all of the articles that CERAD had referenced on its website. Many articles refer to these two papers when they are advancing medical literature related to Alzheimer's disease. A troubling issue in these works is their inclusion in Step 2 (p 481) of age-related changes in the brain tissue samples. Their findings did support my hypothesis of the plaques being caused by small insults to the brain over time. The authors were close to understanding the causes of dementia, but they maintained a belief in the influence of general "brain age," rather than valuing specific insults that brains suffer over time.

$$CCF = CCF_0 - \sum_{n=1}^{N} w_n * f_n(t)$$

$CCF_0 = $ *inital conditions of cognative conscious function*

$N = $ The total number of insults (Example:Micron Strokes) acting in one individual. (Includes the primary and secondary categories)

$w_n = $ *weighing of each risk factor*

$f_n(t) = $ The shape function that describes effect of micron stroke insult, potential recovery as a function of time.

A separate issue is, when excluding dementia from patients without the use of formal neuropsychiatric testing, one must be prepared to miss a significant amount of cognitive dysfunction in the baseline group. Alas, the study would not be a proper study if researchers did not properly exclude those already affected by cognitive problems. A suggested revision for the next CERAD work[xxvii] would be to include complete neuropsychiatric testing on all candidates and to observe all candidates for any of the nine primary factors and over two dozen secondary factors. Then follow their brain tissue in this setting. Normal brain function should be the baseline at the beginning of the study. Following this group over time and closely documenting all of the insults that their brains receive (a.k.a. *micron strokes*) would

---

xxvii   Or whatever organized group takes on such tasks.

provide a good first understanding of how dementia occurs. Once it has been identified and proven how dementia occurs, then one can start prevention of this disease. The cure is possible; **prevention is difficult**.

The National Institutes of Health (NIH) publication[80] is informative, yes, but it starts at a situation of "mild AD" (Alzheimer's disease). The problem is that once you are into mild AD, you are already dreadfully far down that rope and there is not much left for you to hold on to! In fact, the NIH website is full of information that starts where it is already too late for the patient.[81] Prevention of a disease needs to start with an organized plan and evaluation before the disease has taken hold. If you wait for a problem to already be in the mild stages, you will have missed many opportunities of prevention already.

The NIH's list of common changes brought about by "mild Alzheimer's disease" accurately describes people who already have received the diagnosis, but it isn't helpful in determining whether someone has dementia. The following conditions, for example, are so ambiguous they could apply to many people:[82]

- *Loses spark or zest for life; does not start anything*: Sounds like many people I have known. Depression or lack of personal motivation is so pervasive in the population that it would be difficult for a health care provider to see this as medically significant.

- *Loses judgment about money*: The casino must be full of demented people! In the advanced stages of memory disease, people can make strange decisions because of the disease, but I think that one making misjudgments with money is not specific to dementia.

- *Has trouble finding words; may substitute or make up words that sound like or mean something like the forgotten word*: This is considered neologism, Broca's aphasia, and other pathological speech problems. I believe that by the time you develop a problem like this, you cannot be classified as a "mild" of anything. The person affected has had significant insult(s) to the brain once he or she has trouble finding words. As for when "regular folks" grope for a word, you should understand the complex process that occurs inside your brain and the amount of information your brain handles in fractions of a second. Do not fret that your brain feels some lag from time to time. Remember, you are human.[xxviii]

- *Has shorter attention span and less motivation to stay with an activity:* I wonder if the writers of this list have ever been around young adults.

- *Resists change or new things:* This condition sounds like every doctor I have ever met.

- *Has trouble organizing and thinking logically*: Logical thinking is rare. Being organized is a skill that many people work at. Many people spend money to become better organized.

- *Withdraws, loses interest, is irritable; not as sensitive to others' feelings; uncharacteristically angry when frustrated or tired*: I think that this could also describe just about anyone who is employed. That's a bit extreme. But when the economy is bad, many people are irritable and insensitive.

- *Takes longer to do routine chores and becomes upset if rushed or if something unexpected happens:* So does this mean that all of my teenage kids have dementia?

---

xxviii   We would speak for hours on the delicate differences between word finding and memory issues.

- *Forgets to eat, eats only one kind of food, or eats constantly:* Eats constantly? Almost the entire population of the United States fits into this category.

- *Constantly checks, searches, or hoards things of no value:* I watched that *Hoarders* show on TV,[83] and it was something extraordinarily different, but I don't think the people had dementia.

- *Forgets to pay, pays too much, or forgets how to pay— may hand the checkout person a wallet instead of the correct amount of money:* Once I watched a girl at the drive-through of Starbucks pay for her drink and drive off without taking the drink. I asked the employee how often that happens and she responded, "More often than you would believe! Sometimes they will come back around and get the drink, and other times they are just gone!" I am sure the customer I saw didn't have dementia; she just had a lot on her mind and was not concentrating on what she was doing.

The other symptoms listed on the NIH website (such as "asks repetitive questions" and "may stop talking to avoid making mistakes") may genuinely indicate a developing brain disease. But there are so few of these genuine indicators (about five) that it's complicated to make a valid diagnosis of mild dementia without a full neuropsychological evaluation. Assessing the function of the mind without six hours of testing is difficult and a superficial way of treating a patient.

When approaching an evaluation of dementia, everyone is simply guessing because the early indicators can be so subtle that the dedicated time of a full neuropsychiatric evaluation is necessary. I think that the phrase "neuropsychiatric testing" can generate some fear in a patient. I do wish we had a better word for the testing. Explaining it as "Alzheimer's-prevention tests" or "dementia-prevention testing" can make the testing sound less intimidating. If your doctor uses the Mini Mental Status Examination, she is simply wasting your time. This test overlooks meaningful problems, and passing it will give you a false sense of security.

Many current hypotheses of Alzheimer's disease describe brain damage more than they describe the disease. The cholinergic hypothesis includes a deficiency in production of acetylcholine. True, damage brain cells enough, and you will find this deficiency. The tau hypothesis locates the tau protein as the primary factor of neurotoxicity. While the tau hypothesis has been significantly debated, it does not go against my hypothesis. Damage from *micron strokes* in the brain affects a number of cellular, histopathologic, and physiologic responses. The amyloid hypothesis considers that beta amyloid protein disrupts cells in the brain. Although it is not clear how and why the amyloid protein arrives in the brain tissue, this hypothesis works side by side with my hypothesis. Researchers have written papers on the deleterious network hypothesis, which involves free radicals, amyloid protein, metabolism, and calcium. Other thoughts on the etiology of Alzheimer's disease exist, but in all of these you will not find a single verified cause.

When research works toward making breakthroughs for a disease problem, even organized and well-planned studies can trip and fall. I want to briefly review a billion-dollar blunder. Related to the ENHANCE trial a multibillion dollar mistake took place.[84] The related study used data that were not correctly explained. Released in 2008, the study used a unique population (including tobacco users). The trial failed to lower all LDLs below 70 and made a few other mistakes. The researchers monitored carotid arteries for only twenty-four months instead of the five years or more necessary to make a true evaluation. Many of the carotid artery blockages that I have dissolved have required many years of treatment at goal. You cannot expect any significant change in only two years. You might see blockages fail to increase, but actually dissolving them takes a long time. ENHANCE trial data showed a significant decrease in LDL from baseline, but the subjects still had very high cholesterol. When you are shoveling the driveway in the middle of a snowstorm, is nine inches of snow easier to deal with than eleven? You still have a lot of snow. When your LDL is 140, it is still exceedingly high. Yes, it's better than 300, but 140 is still a very high bad cholesterol level. Preventing the original carotid artery stenosis is always going to be much easier than dissolving it. If the researchers could gather those in the study group, eliminate the smoking subjects, remove those with systolic blood pressure over 130, eliminate uncontrolled diabetics, and bring the subjects' LDL to below 70, they would find that they are able to dissolve carotid artery stenosis. For a billion-dollar product, this would be a good option for the company to consider.

The unique population studied in the ENHANCE trial, who had some type of genetic disorder, could also have found that over time they had regression of their carotid artery stenosis, and some of them could even have discovered that there carotids were pristine again. So what really went wrong here that cost billions of dollars in losses?

- The group studied was not typical of the population. To be included, a person needed to have LDL above 210 and genotype-confirmed heterozygous familial hyper-cholesterolemia. If you do not have that genetic disorder, then the data do not apply to you. This is not at all typical of the population who would use these drugs.

- The study did not get LDL to between 50 and 70 but left most at 140+. Although the simvastatin and Zetia group made a very large improvement in LDL, participants still were left with very high cholesterol. How did the authors ever expect that in leaving participants with an LDL above 140 that there would be any improvement in the carotid arteries?

- Some 30 percent of the study group were cigarette smokers, making it quite impossible to gather any useful data about carotid artery conditions.

11

OVARIAN CANCER

If a woman wants to avoid ovarian cancer that spreads, then she needs to monitor and understand the condition of her ovaries. Considering that surviving this cancer is directly linked to the stage a woman is at when diagnosed, no doubt detecting this problem sooner rather than later is a solid advantage. This type of cancer causes 6 percent of cancer deaths in the United States. When dealing with ovarian cancer, a bimanual exam is not sensitive enough to pick up ovarian mass. If a physician tells you differently, then I would like to challenge what he is telling you. If a woman is not at ideal body weight, then evaluating ovarian mass is almost impossible. If a woman finds the exam uncomfortable, then the physician will have to decrease pressure and modify the exam, making it less effective.

When a physician performs a bimanual exam, he or she inserts one or two fingers inside the vagina, and the other hand goes up onto the pelvic skin. The doctor applies pressure with both hands to evaluate the internal organs. The doctor can determine general size and perhaps contours and can locate some areas of pain. But often this pales in comparison to what doctors can learn from a simple ultrasound. Researchers who publish data about looking for signs and symptoms are simply ignoring the problem until it is too late. Researchers who advise against precautionary transvaginal ultrasounds do so for strictly financial reasons. A patient deserves to have the option, cost or no cost, to understand what could be done to prevent the pain and suffering of cancer.

Ovarian cancer comes from a variety of tissues located in the area of the ovaries. Often tumors on the tubes next to the ovaries lead to a diagnosis of ovarian cancer. At times this happens because without detailed information, the pathologist looking at the tissue under the microscope has to give a "best guess." Different types of ovarian cancer include ovarian surface epithelium, mullerian inclusions, endosalpingiosis/endometrioid, clear cell, mucinous, low-grade serous, and fallopian tube mucosa. Fallopian cancer is closely related to ovarian cancer, and, even under the microscope, it is hard to tell if the cancer started in the fallopian tubes or the ovary.

Studies have been completed that prove how often ovarian cancer can be detected and treated early.[85] In this study by Fishman, the ovaries were inspected by ultrasound. When you go for your transvaginal ultrasound, please be sure that the technologists follow the **MPC** Certified criteria[xxix] (and be sure to eliminate uterine and fallopian cancers from your list). You need to walk into your transvaginal ultrasound with a checklist because many ultrasounds are done that do not match the criteria of an **MPC** Certified study. There are no set standards when any ultrasound is completed. Variations in reporting accuracy from facility to facility are great. You will have a difficult

---

xxix   A set of prerequisites and detailed rules that need to be followed as a study is completed and reported. Currently there are no standards as to what your health care team has to report. Thus the **MPC** has demanded necessary details to be sure reports that are **MPC** Certified™ were thorough and complete—or they failed.

time knowing whether the facility doing your testing is being thorough.

A variety of biochemical markers/blood tests relate to problems with the ovaries. An example is the test called CA-125. Papers have been written that study such testing.[86] A few hundred million dollars are spent each year on this lab test. I think this test should be one of the final tests you choose to do. This test is looking for ovarian cancer, perhaps even cancer that has spread. But normal ovaries and some noncancer problems with the ovaries and nearby tissues elevate the level of CA-125 and throw off the test. Between the transvaginal ultrasound and the lab test, the ultrasound is almost always superior. When you walk away from the ultrasound, you are sure about a few organs in that area: bladder, uterus, cervix, fallopian tubes, and ovaries. When you are given a slip of paper with the CA-125 results, you can really be sure only that you do not have ovarian cancer. Worse, the test tells you nothing about the 10 cm precancerous mass in your pelvis. Recall that many cancerous problems start out as precancerous problems.

Most women who are reading this have done nothing to prevent ovarian cancer that spreads. You are getting your medical care by a team that is following current guidelines. The current guidelines are to place you on this pathway: "wait for symptoms, and then get attention." Symptoms are caused by the spreading of the disease, and the person with symptoms has missed her chance to treat the cancer before it spreads.[87] What I suggest to you goes against most guidelines but does not conflict with common sense.

Some experts say that data suggest a patient can still improve when early symptoms are detected. I agree, but good luck in getting a health care team to properly evaluate early symptoms. The health care team will likely treat the patient for muscle sprain, urinary tract infection, ovarian cysts, bloating, or any of the other common symptoms that ovarian cancer can appear to be.

I provide complete gynecological care to all my patients from birth to death. Many recommendations include discontinuing routine health maintenance at a certain age. When one bases recommendations on a patient's age rather than the condition of the patient or the patient's wishes, that health care team is creating psychological abandonment, opening the door for disease to take hold. If the patient is truly able to make the decision—to sit down and watch a video of what dying from uterine cancer or ovarian cancer is like—she may decide that simple, proper medical treatment would be much better.

Often my patients have their own ob-gyn, who at most performs pap smears and sometimes a breast examination. Usually, there is little communication, and the patient is just embarrassed and happy to be done with her ob-gyn visit. Often no one calls her with the results of her testing, and this leaves her with a general idea that "if you hear nothing, everything is okay." This assumption can open a path to destruction.

The uterus and ovaries are *internal* organs, and even if your ob-gyn could find a 5-mm hex nut at the bottom of a bag of nails, it is still difficult on a bimanual examination to determine much other than the fact that the ovaries and uterus are there. Masses the size of golf balls and oranges can easily be hidden or in positions a physician cannot examine. I am sure that there was a point in medicine, before ultrasound machines were available, when the bimanual examination was the most appropriate medical test. But now that we have these tools, we should use them. Ultrasound readings identify structures—normal and abnormal. Abnormal masses, lesions, and tumors would require further evaluation. When properly completed and reported the ultrasound can also take into account the condition of the fallopian tubes, uterus, cervix, and bladder.

I know that there are many physicians, health care providers, and insurance corporations that at this point are saying, "Oh, but what about all of the things that never would have bothered the person," and they're right. Someone with an ovarian mass might well die from something else and never be affected by the mass itself. But until there is some tool or device that can tell such things, I give general advice. Take care of yourself as you did when you were younger, and you will be better situated to see another year. When an ovarian mass is removed, the pathology report may indicate "no cancer"; however, one needs to question how many of those abnormal masses would have become cancerous. Generally, masses over 5 cm should have a higher priority for removal. Follicular cysts and normal process in the ovary can give you smaller cystic structures. The ovary is a very active place, and should you decide to have your health care team order a transvagianal ultrasound—you need to know it will be unique to you on that day. There is simply no way of reporting "normal"—however if completed with details required, you will now know if there is something down there that requires additional attention—or simply check back in a few years.[xxx]

These are the basic steps to preventing metastatic ovarian cancer (which, alarmingly, no one has ever put forth before):

1. At age intervals, perform a **MPC** Certified transvaginal ultrasound. The report from this ultrasound must include specific details, like the careful identification of structures, specific measurements of what is visualized, along with other prerequisites and specific criteria. [xxxi]

2. Anything abnormal or disconcerting is sent off for MRI of the pelvis and affected tissues.

---

xxx   A **MPC** Certified study would result in a passing score for 12-24 months.
xxxi   A long list of criteria and performance prerequisites decreases any low quality reports that would confuse the situation further.

3. The MRI identifies any affected tissues that serves as a baseline, without exposing the patient to radiation.

4. Surgeons, who rarely make mistakes when operating in this area, remove suspected cancerous lesions.

5. Properly trained pathologists document and report on tissues.

You will never receive this treatment unless you ask for or demand it. The simple reason is that it costs your health insurance company more than simply allowing you to get the disease. Do you remember when I explained how pain and suffering is not calculated as a part of cost? Well, this is a perfect example: as calculated by the bean counters, the cost ignores the pain and suffering of coping with cancer—which you can prevent by taking good care of your body.

12

TESTICULAR CANCER

Almost all testicular cancer occurs with a nodule or lump in the testicle. If a man wants to know whether he has testicular cancer, he needs three things: fingers, a thumb, and about fifteen minutes a month. A simple self-examination will pick up any nodules or lesions that a physician is able to pick up. I tell my patients to "spend a TV commercial checking the left boy and right boy." You are going to be much better at it than the physician will. You will be more comfortable, you can spend more time, and you will not be embarrassed. Interestingly enough, physicians are embarrassed when they have to do a testicular examination. However, if your physician is able to move past those embarrassments and provide medical care to you with what I call the "no judgment zone," the same as Planet Fitness, we don't judge. We are here to do our job; we are here to help you. We don't care if you shave or you don't shave. We hope that you have some basic hygiene. However, we don't judge. The patient should feel some degree of hesitancy. If not, then I would actually think there is something wrong with the patient. However, this is a bridge that simply needs to be crossed once a year for most patients and a monthly self-check. Performing that check monthly makes it unlikely that you are going to die from testicular cancer.

It can be embarrassing to have your doctor check on this part of your body or even discuss it with you. This is how it is. That's how our bodies are. We are shy about things, we get embarrassed easily, and we want to remain private. We ignore something and hope that it goes away rather than say, "Oh boy, I should take care of this now rather than later." Lance Armstrong received a diagnosis of testicular cancer in 1996.[88] Presenting symptoms were coughing up blood and testicular swelling to the size of an orange.[89] I have no doubt that organized athletic teams have physicians, but it is unclear whether team physicians bother to check the testicles.

The average age for developing this type of cancer is around thirty-five years old.[90] Men can be at risk their entire lives, but the risk is lower at age eighty-five than at a younger age.

When it comes to testicular cancer, the USPSTF (and others that propose or recommend similar guidelines) really dug into a deep hole. In summary, it "recommends against routine screening for testicular cancer in asymptomatic adolescent and adult males. Grade: D Recommendation."[91] So what that statement means is, "Do not look for testicular cancer. Wait for the day it spreads to your lungs and you spit blood; then go and seek help." The USPSTF went on to explain that "currently most testicular cancers are discovered by patients themselves or their partners, either unintentionally or by self-examination," and that "clinicians should be aware of testicular cancer as a possible diagnosis when young men present to them with suggestive signs and symptoms." I challenge any doctor/clinician to be on his toes enough to keep in mind when a young guy presents with a bit of a cough, that it could be testicular cancer. The required treatment plan in that case—CT scans and X-rays of the chest—

would probably do more harm than good.[xxxii] Most of the testicular cancer and testicular masses that I have diagnosed and cured were still localized to the testicle, and the diagnosis occurred within a week of doing a complete physical.

When USPSTF 2011 evaluated testicular self-examination, it found no studies and no results for mortality, morbidity, or efficacy of the self-exam.[92] I wonder how one can make the jump from something that is not even studied to being able to make a sweeping recommendation. Making a statement such as this is untenable. A proper guideline would simply state: "We do not yet know."

Testicular cancer is an incredibly important cancer that hits younger men who usually do not care much about their health. The youthful feeling of invulnerability makes it even more important to diagnose this cancer before it spreads. Current guidelines indicate that young men should not be checking their testicles. Medical knowledge is that the health care provider, the patients, or their partners notice most testicular cancers. Any suspicious masses can then be further evaluated with ultrasound. Given that most guys have testicles that are readily available for monthly examination, allowing and teaching men to simply check their own testicles each month is a no-brainer. When and if a new mass is noted, then medical attention can be given.

Cryptorchidism is one of the most common risk factors for testicular cancer. This is when a testicle fails to descend into the scrotal sack. As the testicle remains up inside the abdomen, the risk is the highest. An undescended testicle that remains in the inguinal canal also gives elevated rates of cancer. The type of cancer that is identified is also an important part in the treatment plan. One will always do better when this cancer is identified early.

---

xxxii   CT scans and X-ray have radiation exposure and are best used to confirm what you believe to be true.

Differing size between the left and right testicle can sometimes indicate a problem, but it can also simply represent the way you are. You should be suspicious only when the larger testicle continues to grow. Lance Armstrong stated that he had swelling of the testicle for about three years before seeking medical attention.[93] Because his case of metastatic testicular cancer was advanced at the time of diagnosis, it required open brain surgery to remove a tumor from the brain.

13

H E A R T   D I S E A S E

Many of you have a good understanding of how shocking and awful the sudden death of a young athlete can be. Currently, the prevention cardiac care provided to young athletes in the United States is mostly nonexistent. Many of these deaths could be avoided if doctors advise a plan with an electrocardiogram (EKG) in it. Simply doing an EKG might have prevented what you read about in the news periodically. At a national conference once, I told my friend how we should be running presport EKGs for young athletes rather than just simply assuming that all is normal. The next day he said to me, "Hey, did you see the news last night? A kid collapsed on the basketball court. Dead." If only his doctor had offered an EKG, that sad situation might have been averted.

For a test that costs $9.71 in 2012,[xxxiii] simply hooking the EKG[xxxiv] machine onto the kids and letting the computer do its interpre-

---

xxxiii   Reimbursement for obtaining the EKG tracing by Medicare.
xxxiv   The EKG is a when a computer detects the electrical currents that run in the heart and evaluate them for a pattern.

tation would be better than doing nothing at all. Any abnormal readings can be sent on for further evaluation. Every school could consider this, and then spend more funds on having physicians read over tests to further improve accuracy. Completing an EKG and an echo would effectively approve a young athlete for a vigorous sport. Other authors have reviewed the lack of proper attention to our athletic young.[94]

To further reduce risk, the athlete can pass a treadmill stress test with imaging. For this test you need to have someone who would almost be overqualified for the job. When doctors are looking for disease that is rare, they need to perform the test with great sensitivity. A confusing aspect of medical testing is that often a patient passes a stress test with flying colors yet still has significant blockages in the coronary arteries. I am sure there isn't much evidence to support the cost of such testing, but for the rare young adult who turns out to be at risk, I am sure the family would prefer the option of testing. Here we are again—the least expensive test is the one that makes the diagnosis. Luckily, on the topic of preventing sudden cardiac death in young athletes, blockages of the coronary arteries are going to be rare, and the evaluation of the electrical system will clearly identify more of the asymptomatic problems.

Are these families ever given a choice? Does the health care team sit down with them and explain that a series of simple tests can eliminate the risk of some significant problems? I suspect not. Does anyone explain that some rare diseases are discovered only with an invasive catheterization? And that some diseases are discovered only at autopsy?[xxxv]

Playing sports is simple. If an athlete has no symptoms, then perhaps he can just take a chance by not knowing his body. But if the athlete has a cardiac murmur or chest pain, has ever passed out, or if his family history includes conditions like this, the youngster should get tested and smile nicely at the health

---

xxxv   Solitary coronary artery.

care provider who says it isn't necessary. Some might have access to a "sports physical." Most doctors give the preparticipation sports physicals in such a superficial and limited way that they constitute nothing more than signing off on a form. I think 99 percent of the effort should be spent on preventing sudden cardiac death. Most orthopedic conditions will be symptomatic and independently evaluated by the athlete or parents.

A rope company tests the strength of every type of rope before it sends it out to a customer. Why is it standard to check the strength of a rope before selling it but not to check the heart of a child who will engage in competitive sports? I know that my line of thinking will meet with a significant amount of resistance from people who want "positive predictive factors" and statistics. Those people can refer to my other section where I discuss the significance and insignificance of statistics. Yes, they are important and sometimes helpful, but the pain and suffering of the family who suddenly loses a child supersedes any of the statistics someone can show to me. Some health care teams will rely more on the power of statistics than on preventing medical conditions, but most families would rather pay for an EKG than bury a loved one.

In over a decade of treating people, I am still amazed at how often the symptoms of heart disease are silent. Once looked for, heart disease shows its ugly head easily, but when allowed to do its own thing, it destroys you. Most people feel relatively fine at the time of diagnosis of heart disease. When we discover heart disease without symptoms, we have time to fix and treat the problems.

If your health care team follows current guidelines, then it is unlikely that the team has given much attention to your heart. Your doctor will tell you how to reduce your risk of heart disease, but you need to realize that most of the things that your health care team tells you are not very effective. Ask your doctor how much "changing your ways" will help. If he is a quality physician, he will tell you that he doesn't know and that there's a chance that changing your behavior won't help much.[95] Don't get me wrong—changing your behavior probably won't hurt, but it may not help. Challenge your health care team: ask what the condition of your mitral valve is or the size of your left atrium. I wonder what your conversation will be after you ask that question.

BICUSPID AORTIC VALVE: Heart disease killed more than six hundred thousand people in 2006. More than 25 percent of the deaths in the United States are caused by heart disease.[96] One in fifty people has a bicuspid aortic valve, a medical condition for which sudden death is the only warning sign. Yes, this common problem is mostly ignored. A bicuspid aortic valve is one with only two cusps rather than the usual three. The valve opens and closes about a hundred and ten thousand times a day. (You don't often find anything that man has made that can stand up to that type of wear and tear. Your maker did a good job when he designed the valve, no matter what version you have inside your chest.) Because blood has to flow differently, and the valve ends up contacting across a different physical pattern, it wears out quickly. By age forty-five, people with a bicuspid aortic valve have already developed a significant problem but may be unaware of it.

You can save your life by simply knowing what type of valve you have. If you have a bicuspid aortic valve—which can run in families—then you should pay attention to it. A 2-D echo that is **MPC** Certified will allow you to know. Unfortunately for most people, when they go for a 2-D echo, it is unlikely that a doctor will read the report for the correct details. At times the tech who collects the data is not experienced. Other times the doctor who reads the report spends only a fraction of the time that should be spent and reports a superficial description.[97] Generally, by about age eleven, there is already wear and tear on the heart valves that can be detected. If the group reading your 2-D echoes is conscientious enough to report the small leaks and wear on the valves, then you might be in a good situation. Much of the data you get will also serve as baseline data for the condition of your valves.

I treated a patient once who came from the Midwest. She had just moved to my town. While in her Midwest town, she had a cardiac catheterization because of chest pain and was found to have a critical 50 percent LAD lesion. The advice to the patient was to undergo semiurgent coronary artery bypass surgery. She refused. She moved out to my state, and I picked her up as a patient. The first two pounds of her paper chart were related to the discussions of her critical coronary artery disease. We reviewed multiple times the advice of other physicians who were involved with her care, advice that the patient adamantly refused. Given the cowboy nature of this patient's plan[xxxvi], reviewed medical literature at that time suggested that a lower LDL is better. She was able to take 40 mg of Lipitor, and her LDL remained in the range of 40–60 for many years. She also worked with diet and exercise as a backup to the medication. Four to five years later, she again developed chest pain. This time she was quite concerned, and she wanted an evaluation. Because of her prior diagnosis, her first desire was to go back to the cardiac cath lab. Findings at the time of the cardiac cath were significant for clean coronaries, pristine. Yes, she was able to dissolve her prior blockages. After three more tests—ultrasound of the gallbladder, Hida scan, and an EGD—the patient's diagnosis was a bad gallbladder. She underwent uneventful laparoscopic cholecystectomy. After her cholecystectomy, her pain and symptoms resolved, leaving a happy and appreciative patient.

This situation set in my mind the importance of LDL levels and the possibility of actually dissolving blockages. To this date, current medical literature that follows blockages (such as the ENHANCE trial)[98] monitor only over two years.

---

xxxvi   A plan that throws much caution to the wind, holds on tight, and sees what happens next.

You have blood vessels, which are called arteries. Each of your arteries is made up of two types of cells: smooth muscle cells and endothelial cells. A replication of the cellular DNA without division into new cells can happen in the arterial muscle fibers as a response to high blood pressure.[99] If you cut a blood vessel in half, you would notice that there are many layers of the smooth muscle cells. As some of the blood vessels get even larger and have dozens of layers of smooth muscle cells, they get their own blood supply (vasa vasorum).

Generally, blood flows at a low rate and at high pressure; once in the capillaries, it flows at a higher rate but at a lower pressure. Capillary pressure is important because if it is increased, then certain proteins are pushed out of the blood into the interstitial tissue. If you change the pressure of the capillaries, you are changing many things in the environment of the capillary. You change so many things that current science has no idea of what is happening. Hypertension can be caused by many things: sodium transport, peripheral resistance, renin-angiotensin, renal function, cardiac output, body position, stresses, renal artery stenosis, aldosterone secretion, blood flows, blood viscosity, endothelial cell responses, various mineralcorticoids, changes in the sympathetic nervous system outputs, end organ effects, and others. When the kidney wants blood, it will get blood! Many other factors—such as brain natriuretic peptide, pain, medications, and dietary changes—are also involved. Clearly, there is no simple or obvious explanation for what causes any given case of hypertension. You could more easily enumerate the individual brush strokes that make up the Mona Lisa. But make no mistake—hypertension and atherosclerosis are closely linked. If you do not respect them and treat them, your doom awaits.

Many current recommendations involve waiting on new data, and while we're all waiting for more data, heart disease is still the number one killer in the United States. Many victims have plenty of warning and plenty of opportunity for early medical intervention. But for many others (several hundred thousand a year), sudden death is the first sign that anything is wrong. So it is incredibly reasonable for Americans to wonder about the state of their coronary arteries, even if they're feeling entirely well.

The USPSTF, as usual, recommended against screening—with resting electrocardiography (ECG), exercise treadmill test (ETT), or electron-beam computerized tomography (EBCT) scanning for coronary calcium in any risk group. This recommendation is incomprehensible in light of the amount of cardiac disease that exists.[100] Simply put, with how much heart disease exists, more should be done in prevention. I do not put EBCT high on my list, as many coronary problems can still be missed and you need radiation exposure.

Currently, there is no completely accepted definition for hypertension. Organizations offer different values for what your blood pressure should or should not be. I say the number is 119.

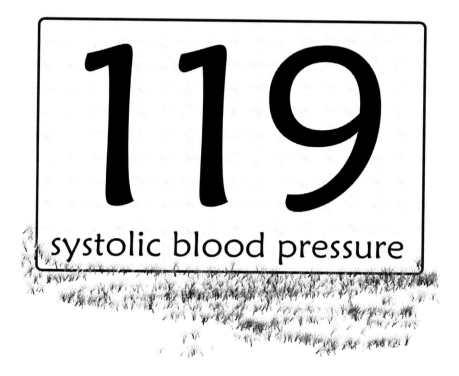

119 systolic blood pressure

See that number? Don't ever let your blood pressure be above that number. That is what your body feels at the max limit. The kidney and hypertension are linked like peanut butter and jelly. A doctor who specializes in the function of the kidney, a nephrologist, will tell you that although we know much about the kidney, there are volumes of data we don't understand. Do not confuse your mind with terms such as *"borderline," "benign," "severe," "malignant"*—let's just keep things simple! Either you have hypertension or you don't. There is no predisease. Do not shirk your task of lifelong blood pressure control by slipping into a classification that allows damage to take place. Either you have been taking care of your problem or you just discovered it. It is possible that you have had hypertension for years and it has done damage to your body, or it is new and your organs have not yet paid the price. Any textbook that reviews renal vascular disease will explain how the disease of the kidney at the glomerular level is different from other types of renal disease. When it comes to the hypertensive destruction of the kidney, you will find normal and abnormal glomeruli right next to each other.

High blood pressure costs over $70 billion a year.[101] Management of high blood pressure in the United States is based upon guidelines. The Joint National Committee (JNC) has completed many of the guidelines. The guidelines have changed over the years but have never simply set a systolic blood pressure limit of 120. There is no disadvantage, given current medications and treatments on the market today, to capture and treat all of the hypertension that requires medical management. Many of the medications have additional benefits for many organs (heart valves, kidneys, pancreas). Page 11 of JNC 6, archived, year 1997, indicates that optimal blood pressure is lower than 120. Why is there so much confusion? If your systolic blood pressure is above 120, then you have high blood pressure. The higher it goes the worse that it is for your organs. JNC 6 and the JNC reviews since 1976 have led to JNC 7. The World Health Organization[102] and JNC 7 start with a systolic blood pressure of 140 as your threshold. With JNC 7, a predisease is added, "prehypertension." How sad, because you cannot have a pre-disease. You either have a medical condition or you do not.

Less than 50 percent of hypertensive patients have their blood pressure under control.[103] When one considers the more than forty million who have a systolic blood pressure between 120 and 139, then the number of properly treated patients dwindles to a small fraction. A systolic blood pressure of 138 will get you a pat on the back from JNC 7. I have a nephrologist friend who brags about the D.A.S.H diet. He is wicked smart, so you should be sure to know and understand this diet. The D.A.S.H diet is inexpensive. (Visit the NIH or dashdiet.org for more information.)

Often advice from an academy on how to care for your heart is based upon some type of medical research. As you are unique, you may not match the population that was involved with the research. However, you might be blended into the guidelines and conclusions that result. Many readers of this section are fa-miliar with the ACCORD study.[104] If you are curious about your primary cardiovascular outcome or rate of death from any cause—specifically rates of stroke and nonfatal stroke—then follow its published advice. Be sure that you also have type 2 diabetes if you wish to apply their findings. If this doesn't apply to you, keep the number 119 in mind.

The ACCORD study is no doubt a well-constructed study, and a significant amount of effort was completed. But the conclusions from ACCORD should be restricted to the group that was stud-ied. The study covered too many different aspects to gather complete unique patient data. The authors included ten thou-sand high-risk participants with type 2 diabetes mellitus. The par-ticipants were divided into a variety of groups, including some who received multiple cholesterol treatment drugs, some who received intensive or standard treatment of their diabetes, and some who received a placebo. But including current and for-mer cigarette-smoking participants clearly skewed the results of the study. You simply can't include cigarette smoking and accurately evaluate for reduction in stroke-type events—it will not happen. Those who smoke will have strokes and cardiac events. The results apply only to the specific population that was studied (cigarette-smoking diabetics with high blood pressure and high cholesterol) and are simply inaccurate for anyone outside that population.

When a child has a heart murmur, doctors should check a 2-D echo. New technology allows some providers to even check the heart valves in the office, but it will take years for that to become common practice. The idea of using Doppler and ultrasound to evaluate the heart rather than a stethoscope can be compared to completing a laparoscopic cholecystectomy versus an open cholecystectomy. Not everyone would go to a surgeon who only did open cases. Most would want the "bellybutton surgery." Same could be said for a provider who uses a stethoscope to diagnose a cardiac murmur in a child. Given that bicuspid aortic valve is common, why would a provider ignore a heart murmur? The best pediatric cardiologist listens to the heart, does the 2-D check, and verifies the findings. With a 2-D echo, the patient receives no radiation, and the TV screen shows the valves and flow and whether the plumbing is hooked up right and there are no leaks. This simple test enables the doctor to diagnose either a significant cardiac problem or a condition that can be monitored over time with future 2-D echo.

Most pediatric cardiologists who are practicing health care (and psychological abandonment) suggest that no echoes should be done or ordered for follow-up. You and your child deserve better. You deserve to know the condition of the cardiac chambers and of the heart valves. Remember that bicuspid aortic valves often won't make themselves known until the patient suddenly dies. Many pediatric and adult cardiologists attempt to "conserve resources" in blindfolded support for insurance company profits rather than doing what they should by their profession.

Consider some doctors who use the stethoscope to determine nebulous sounds of the heart and what they could mean. To be clear, part of medical school and residency involves developing a critical understanding of the specific heart sounds—decreased intensity of S1 could be a severely calcified mitral valve; increased S1 intensity could be mitral stenosis; and other sounds. Persistently split S2, paradoxically split, fixed split S2, soft P2, for example, are all crucial to understanding the physiology of the heart. I would definitely state that for the education of health care providers, or anyone who is in the study of medicine, that they understand all those terms. A good physician understands how anatomy and physiology change with different predicted sounds of the heart, but it is not a very good physician who uses his stethoscope as the final call. There is simply not enough accuracy in the use of the stethoscope when determining the disease state of the heart.

With the amount of heart disease in the world, my statement is proven correct. Perhaps if more people had 2-D echo information, then concerned health care teams would know what they are dealing with. A 2-D echo identifies multiple things—pressures, valves, pump function, structure, and anatomy—easily and without risk to the patient. The stethoscope, my favorite health care tool, is antiquated. A 2-D echo of the heart is my favorite medical tool. I pose this question to health care providers: Why are you guessing as you treat your patients? I have no idea why children and young adults are not afforded the chance to know the condition of their heart valves before they reach an age when the damage is permanent.

But before you run out for a 2-D echo of your heart, you should be aware of a few things. Many echo reports are read inaccurately and without attention to the details. They receive a quick glance, and the vital information is not recorded. Make sure some reads your 2-D echo carefully and completely. An early focus group reviewer of this work wanted to know how, as a patient, she could be sure her study is completed properly. The **MPC** has a long list of criteria and prerequisites that go into the proper reporting of a 2-D echo study. We constantly adjust the list with additional details as technology changes and more physicians are qualified to do such detailed work. You can contact the **MPC** if you have nowhere else to turn, are motivated, and really need that type of help. As for the answer to my focus group member, we discussed a bit of news that occurred in 2010 when a New York hospital was routinely skipping the physician interpretation. As the news reported, a technician completed the studies, but a physician read them only if the technician believed there was something abnormal.[105] When the health care world that you are living in allows such events to take place, other than offering a **MPC** Certified study to this member, there was no accurate way to be sure the work was completed and reported properly without guessing.

Regardless of which path you decide to take, understanding the condition of your heart valves will give you about five years of heads up to make simple adjustments to medications and monitor your condition. The naysayers will lament the associated costs and expenses, but I have clearly stated that the least expensive test is the one that makes the diagnosis. Period. End of the discussion from me. Do the test. Make the diagnosis. I find it rare that after age eleven a heart murmur cannot be detected. Yes—eleven years old. When children reach age eleven their hearts have beaten approximately 445,665,000 times—the valves bashing on each other. Wear and tear has already started. Does every child at age eleven *need* an echo? I didn't say that. But I can assure anyone who has never had an echo the **MPC** would identify what you need to know about the condition of your heart valves. Then your health care team or even Google could help you understand what you need to do to prevent further damage.[xxxvii]

---

xxxvii   Your needs and what treatment would be best are unique to you, beyond the scope of this chapter.

14

THYROID/PANCREAS/LIVER/ KIDNEY/ GALLBLADDER/OTHER DISEASES

Thyroid

What are you doing to prevent thyroid cancer from spreading? In a thirty-year study, only 2 of 140 thyroid cancers were detectable by physical examination.[106] Thyroid cancer accounts for forty-four thousand new cases and one thousand deaths in the United States each year.[107] Common screening tests are ultrasound and a neck exam.[108]

Ultrasound of thyroid

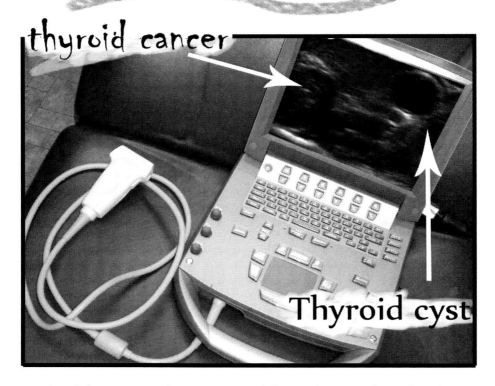

thyroid cancer

Thyroid cyst

In this example one would not know they had a thyroid cancer without the use of the ultrasound.

A thyroid cyst can be found commonly when ultrasound is used.

On a physical examination, one or both could be missed, and cyst or solid cancer would never be known.

Physical examination of the thyroid is extremely difficult because the thyroid can blend right in with many other normal structures in the neck. So what this tells you is that when you go to your health care provider for evaluation of thyroid cancer, the only thing that hands on your neck do is make you feel better. Hands on your neck will not be able to determine whether you have a cancer. Most neck surgeons would concur that once they cut into the neck, structures appear that are difficult to detect with their hands. Physicians who do twenty or thirty neck exams per day might be more skilled than those who do fewer, but without an ultrasound of your thyroid, you really have no idea of its exact contour. Masses of the thyroid do not cause any symptoms until they grow to a significant size. You simply do not know whether you have thyroid cancer. The simple ultrasound identifies size, configuration, and presence of masses. Knowing this is better than not knowing this.

Task force recommendations and guidelines, once again, state that no studies have yielded evidence that finding a thyroid cancer before it spreads is of any benefit. But no one has ever conducted a study on that kind of prevention specifically, and simply because a subject has not been studied does not mean that it isn't valid or valuable. Finding any cancer before it spreads is always beneficial.[xxxviii] Palpation of your neck by anyone in your health care team amounts to a superficial level of care, unless you have a large mass or goiter. Biopsy is required for any suspicious findings. Without a biopsy doctors have a difficult time diagnosing a cancer. No clinical benefits of any type of screening have been either studied or established. I insist that knowing the configuration of your thyroid, and whether there are nodules over 10 mm in size, is a drastic improvement over not knowing at all. We can diagnose and cure thyroid cancer. (Some doctors will raise concern over the risk of complication at the time of the biopsy, but to me that does not mean the biopsy

---

xxxviii   Often complete surgical removal of thyroid cancer requires no further treatments. Metastatic thyroid cancer requires additional treatments along with the surgery.

is a bad idea. If you need work done, then get it done, and be sure that whoever is coming at you with a knife or needle knows what he is doing.)

The American Association of Clinical Endocrinologists (AACE) and the American College of Endocrinology (ACE) have published their plans for managing thyroid carcinoma.[109] They stated that thyroid cancer is the "forgotten cancer" and is responsible for more deaths than all other endocrine cancers combined. Unfortunately, as with most published information, there is no recommended plan for the prevention of thyroid cancer that spreads. The key recommendation from 2010 AACE publications is, "Ultrasound evaluation is not recommended as a screening test in the general population."[110] This puts you in a difficult situation. Everyone will tell you that picking up your thyroid cancer before it spreads is close to impossible without doing an ultrasound. But no one will tell you to go and get an ultrasound of your thyroid. I guess that is my job here. Go get an ultrasound of your thyroid and understand what that organ is doing. Following current guidelines and waiting for a swollen lymph node to appear could result in unpleasant cancer treatment. You should take charge of your health and understand your body.

For clarity lab work will not detect thyroid cancer—only locating and evaluating the tissue of your thyroid can do that. Many readers may have had a thyroid-stimulating hormone test (TSH) as part of lab work.[xxxix] When your TSH is normal, or needs medical attention, you understand the function of that gland, but this is not related to thyroid cancer. A normal TSH means that the gland is functioning properly (or you are taking your medications properly), but the gland has not been completely evaluated with only lab data.

---

xxxix   Thyroid-stimulating hormone, released in the brain to instruct the thyroid gland in the neck how to behave.

The Pancreas and Other

Pancreatic cancer is often called a "silent killer" because it can spread before it presents any noticeable problems. Understanding the configuration of your pancreas will put you on your way to preventing your death from metastatic pancreatic cancer. (As is the case for many organs, you will go far and wide before you find another health care professional telling you to be sure to understand your pancreas.)

In 2011 Steve Jobs, the CEO of Apple, died from pancreatic cancer.[111] The information available indicates pancreatic cancer and a liver transplant. Neither Jobs nor Patrick Swayze, who also died from pancreatic cancer, had any practical limitations on what they could spend on health care or medical care. Both of these individuals, if they simply had an MRI of the pancreas at any time during the years before the disease worsened, no doubt could have improved their condition. I am not trying to explain that pancreatic cancer could have been totally prevented; rather, what could have been prevented is the spreading of that cancer.

The mini-Whipple is a surgical procedure performed at Thomas Jefferson Hospital in Philadelphia. Cure is possible in cases of pancreatic cancer that have not yet spread (and even precancerous lesions). Often this surgical procedure cures a patient from pancreatic cancer. I do not think it's a matter of individuals not wanting to prevent the disease. Rather, it is more likely they are just simply unaware. When identified early, pancreatic cancer can be removed and no chemotherapy will be required.[xl]

---

xl   Be sure you REALLY know all of the details and risks and benefits by talking with a cancer specialist (oncologist), as this type of data changes very often, and you need always to be treated with the most updated science.

Division of Cancer cell

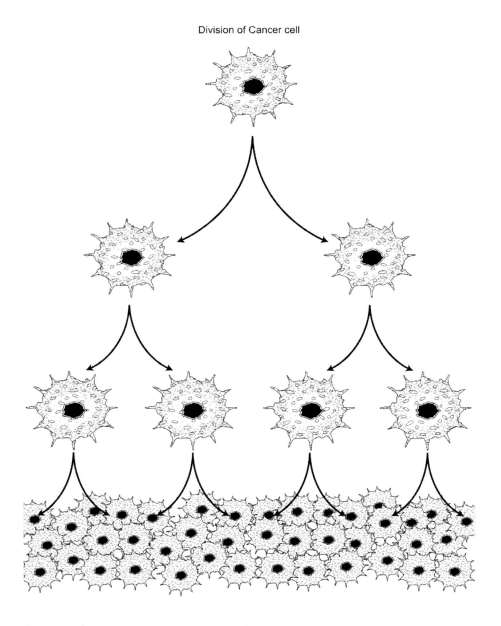

Remember, cancer starts as a single messed-up cell. This cell divides and multiplies. Once a certain mass of cells has grown, the cancer can enter the blood stream and become metastatic. Your body attempts to recognize and wall off these abnormal cells. As the mass of cells grows, it reaches a size that ultrasound or other imaging can detect. Removing the mass when it was in the body but hadn't yet spread would have prevented the disease state in both of these respected men.

Imaging of the pancreas can be a bit more difficult than imaging some of the other organs because of a few unique factors. If you are overweight, ultrasound of your abdomen is more difficult. There are multiple ways to get images of the pancreas, each with individual risks and results. MRI and ultrasound are two of my favorite ways to evaluate an organ because there is no radiation involved. Someday 9.4 Tesla MRI scans could be widely available, helping you identify the condition of your pancreas.

These tests can illuminate vital information about other organs, too—the liver, kidneys, adrenal glands, and gallbladder. Give some attention to your kidneys every few years, and you will not die from metastatic kidney cancer. A health care team can have a hard time distinguishing a precancerous polyp from a gallstone. (If you do have a polyp in your gallbladder, spend a morning and have it removed. Laparoscopic cholecystectomy is an outpatient procedure that removes the gallbladder, and most people go home the same day.)

Other rare types of cancers that I have not been able to successfully integrate into the **MPC** include some types of bone cancers. For these the best advice is that whenever you or your loved one has persistent pain,[xli] have it evaluated. Because often pain can be referred from nearby joints, I recommend getting X-rays of the joints both above and below the pained area. Without asking for X-rays of the nearby joints, it is quite likely that you will get an X-ray of only the affected area. Avoid radiation if you can. But in consideration of a cancer or tumor, an X-ray is appropriate and will definitely be worth your time and effort.

---

xli   Not a one-time sore limb or joint after soccer games.

People often have abnormal blood clots. Many blood specialists and hematologists across the United States do not want these people further evaluated. Rather, they wait for the second event to take place. Sadly, if the first or second event is not severe enough to be detected, then neither is evaluated. I doubt that most blood specialists even understand how to complete a thorough evaluation. The **MPC** has a complete list of what should be evaluated in light of a clotting disorder. When I order the hypercoagulable evaluation for a patient, the profile is detailed and comprehensive. Blood clots also include complete evaluation of current active cancer, a bit overwhelming for an already stressed health care team; however, for a physician of medicine very rewarding results.

All through medical school and residency, I encountered a variety of options for evaluation of an individual with a blood clot or clotting disorder. Few reference books are complete. I am sure that throughout the United States, many blood specialists complete hypercoagulable evaluations for adult and pediatric patients and truncate some of those evaluations. Often I find that outside testing by a specialist is only for a Factor V Leiden. It's unclear why a specialist would shortchange patients like this. I guarantee that happens over and over again. If you are a hematologist who actually does a thorough and complete hypercoagulable workup on your patients, then I am confident that you will appreciate how difficult it is for you to get those around you to understand what to do. Factor V Leiden is an inherited blood disorder that increases blood clot risks. David Bloom, the NBC News correspondent, died in 2003 from a blood clot in his leg moving up into his lung. Many cramped days and nights inside army vehicles is a risk factor in the development of a blood clot in the leg.

The proper evaluation is simple—up to fourteen vials of blood, when you come right down to it. (Drink an extra glass or two of water before you go for your labs.) What those vials reveal will prevent a stroke, pulmonary embolism, or future dementia.

They also shed light on the health of your children and perhaps even your parents. Blood disorders are genetic, so once an individual receives a diagnosis, it opens up the ability for the entire family to understand what is happening. Parents' blood work will save children. Factor V and Factor II gene mutations identified in a parent can be applied to the daughter and can make the difference between life and death for that girl. Decisions on the use of oral contraception need to include the significant amount of risk.[xlii]

I have had many patients over the years who, when properly treated for these hypercoagulable states, were able to give birth to beautiful, normal children. Before undergoing the detailed evaluation, they were fraught with multiple miscarriages and no answers. Doctors brushed off and patted many of them on the back. People deserve better. When you have a medical event, you deserve specific answers. If the answers are not readily available, or if obtaining them requires a significant amount of pain and suffering, then I understand why you would avoid them. But if your answers were just a lab stop away, why would you avoid understanding yourself? Some readers might know of a woman trying to have a baby and who is distraught by recurrent miscarriages without any answers. I hope that you now have a better understanding that so much more can be done to help the situation!

When you are not provided the opportunity to understand your body, then you have no chance for prevention. And let me be clear—I am talking about a *noninvasive* opportunity for you to understand what is happening with your body. In the examples I have given on pancreatic problems, both of these individuals possibly could have purchased a portable ultrasound machine and had a qualified technicians fly out to their house to perform a complete evaluation. Not everyone has the financial

---

xlii   Hormone manipulation will also cause coagulation problems, and when stacked on top of preexisting coagulation problems, the usually safe use becomes a topic for a very deep discussion.

freedom of house calls for Medical Prevention, but you should be aware the cure is possible.

Checking routine labs and monitoring for enlarged lymph nodes that do not go away over time are the best ways to evaluate lymphomas. Do not get excited about single lymph nodes that come about with an infection, as these are your body's routine way of dealing with infection and the immunity process. But if a lymph node becomes significantly enlarged—the size of an egg yolk or larger—or if it does not go away after six weeks, then you should seek further evaluation.

15

COLON AND STOMACH CANCERS

The third most common cause of death in men and women is colorectal. This is a preventable disease. When people consider colon cancer, they should also think of rectal, stomach, and esophageal cancers. When doctors evaluate for these types of cancers, they use a scope to do it the right way. Getting a scope through your colon and down into your stomach every few years will keep away the grim reaper. The scope can find polyps and conditions that are relatively easy to identify and treat. Doctors can remove polyps and treat infections and irritation from acid and acid reflux, preventing cancer from starting. Considering all of the gastrointestinal diseases that can be prevented before age fifty, one cannot fathom why anyone would wait till age fifty. Haters at this point will start to discuss how there are no data to suggest that removing polyps at a younger age is of any long-term benefit. But they have to admit that colon cancers often start in a polyp, and that removing polyps from the colon decreases the risk of cancer.

Many published medical articles agree that removing pre-cancerous polyps from your colon prevents colon cancer. So get into the hands of a GI specialist who does colonoscopies all day long, and get your colonoscopy. Get one every few years. If your health care team is following current guidelines, then your team will check you for colon cancer only from age fifty through seventy-five.[112] Many cancers of the colon happen before age fifty. You need to consider what you are doing to prevent gastrointestinal cancers.

I agree that newer fecal occult blood cards are a big help. They help because when a patient does the card, any blood found will generate an evaluation of the GI system for that patient. However, many cancers are found in spite of normal occult blood cards. Our technology simply isn't perfected enough to detect bleeding from every precancerous or cancerous polyp. Having properly performed scopes of your GI system is a good way for you to sleep at night.

However, many of the scope procedures are inaccurate. When you go for your scope, make sure that the data collected meets specific criteria. The "withdraw time" of the scope, experience of the operator, number of cases completed each day, and where the pathology goes to be reviewed are all important factors. When a prep done by a patient is not adequate, the GI specialist should repeat the study the following day.[xliii] (If your prep is inadequate, how could you expect the specialist to see anything?)

Over the years, I have had a certain rare situation that is difficult. A less-than-adequate operator performed a colonoscopy, and a few months later the patient had an episode of rectal bleeding. If one of the thorough consultations that I use did not com-

---

xliii   For a colon prep, you need to drink a medicated clear liquid, and hours later what comes out of you would start to be as clear as the liquid you are drinking—that would be a good prep. There are other options also, but usually the good old jug of liquid prepares your colon the best for the scope procedure.

plete the initial scope, I insist that the scope be repeated. Too often when the scope is repeated (at times just a few months after the initial scope) we find a big problem—a large polyp or even a golf–ball-sized cancerous mass, which goes to show that your scope needs to be done in a conscientious way, with attention to many details in each step of the process.

16

BREAST CANCER

To prevent breast cancer from spreading, you need to identify it before it spreads. An excellent approach to preventing cancer from spreading is to identify and remove it while it is a solitary mass.

Recall that many current guidelines allow you to fall through the cracks. Task force recommendations for patients older than seventy-five basically resign them to having cancer spread through their bodies. A known fact is that the number one risk factor for breast cancer is increase in age, so why would you avoid detecting breast cancer when you are most at risk? If you are in poor health or are ready for the glue factory, I can understand why you give up on prevention. But most people at age seventy-five are doing okay, so why give up? Worse, why do health care teams give up on them? Those questions need to be understood.

A painless mass detected in your breast could be a cancer. Self-examination is an excellent way for you to understand what is happening in your breast. If you pick up an abnormal mass, have it evaluated. MRI of the breast is a good way to assess a breast mass that could be trouble. One could write an entire book on all of the aspects of what could happen once you detect a mass in your breast. As I have discussed in this work, be sure that anyone working on you has a good understanding of breast mass. A typical issue that many guidelines underscore is that even if a mass is noncancerous, you might feel anxiety. This is when you need to choose how you want to care for your body. Men are not out of the woods on this problem either. Men get breast cancer also. Men and women should know and understand breast tissue. Get a good evaluation of any abnormal lumps that you, your partner, or your health care provider detects. Some breast cancer can be noted simply by looking at the skin of the breast. Dimpling, discharge, or abnormal skin textures can indicate a problem of the breast tissue related to a deeper problem. Breast self-examination is free and simple.

Men and women get breast cancer, so be sure to know and understand your own body.

I have included additional issues about breast cancer in the section that reviews the current guidelines driving your health care team.

Many residents at assisted-living facilities, spending anywhere from $1000 to $10000 per month for their food and shelter, live with medical problems that will bring severe pain and suffering to their lives. How simple it would be to cure that breast cancer before it becomes metastatic. I have done this. I have done this many times for people in such facilities.[xliv] They deserve that quality of life. They deserve to be able to pass from this world without the undue pain and suffering that metastatic breast cancer brings with it—spreading to the brain, filling the lungs with fluid, and making breathing extremely difficult or im-

---

xliv   Simply taking care of a breast lump before the cancer spreads. Allowing for a relatively simple treatment plan that will last for decades.

possible. When a cancer advances like this, the patient spends much time and energy undergoing radiation therapy to alleviate some of the lesions. It is called a palliative measure, but it is essentially defensive. Once the cancer is metastatic, the chance for a cure greatly diminishes. The time for you and your loved ones is *now*! Prevent it now; prevent the pain and suffering. The cure is possible; prevention is difficult, but you can do it. I have told you this already, and I know that you can.

17

P R O S T A T E   C A N C E R

Prostate cancer is the number one killer of men, yet there is not an adequate plan to detect and treat it in the age group that is most at risk. If your health care team follows current guidelines, and you are a man over age seventy-five, then you better be prepared. You are at the age of highest risk, yet no one is doing anything for you. If you are a man younger than age seventy-five looking to your health care team for advice, you will also have a difficult time. The USPSTF concluded, "The current evidence is insufficient to assess the balance of benefits and harms of prostate cancer screening in men younger than age 75." It also recommended against screening for prostate cancer in men age seventy-five years and older. This leaves men in a difficult position, as no matter what their age, they have no advice.

Understand that if you are a male over forty, you are at risk for prostate cancer. Get a rectal exam and do a PSA—prostate-specific antigen. The PSA test comes with a reference range. If the number is in the reference range, that is generally a good thing.[xlv] The PSA test can be elevated in cases of enlargement, infection, and cancer. If the PSA is elevated and you do not have any symptoms of either enlargement or infection of the prostate, then you have a problem. When you find your lab data or examination has become abnormal, get further evaluation. There needs to be a coordination of the health care team's examination of your prostate along with the lab data. Ultrasound or MRI of the prostate can help further define your problem. I have had cases in which the MRI of the prostate, although a technology that most urologists seem to resist in making the diagnosis of prostate cancer, has assisted the diagnosis by pointing to the area of the prostate where cancer was.

Most of my new adult male patients have never had a digital rectal exam. Some current recommendations even seem to cloud the issue of doing a simple manual prostate exam in men at risk of prostate cancer. True, the doctor can feel only part of the gland on examination, and any part of the gland can get cancer. But manual examination is far better than none at all and is a valuable safeguard, considering some cases of prostate cancer and nodules have a normal PSA. I have diagnosed many prostate cancers in my patients because of simple attention to the tissue that is at risk of cancer.

Treatment options once the cancer is diagnosed are beyond the scope of this work. However, you will be in a better position knowing you have a cancer that has an expected clinical course. The prostate cancer grows inside the prostate. Then it gets into the tissue outside of the prostate (capsule). Finally, the prostate cancer will get into the blood and lymph tissue. Once in the blood stream, the prostate cancer finds its way to bones, lungs, and liver. Taking care of one patient who has to die from metastatic prostate cancer is enough for any conscientious physician to want to avoid that clinical situation. Dying from

---

xlv   Rarely an increase in number over years, but still in reference range, can also indicate problems. (Example: 2013 result 1.2, 2014 result 1.3, 2015 result 4.1.)

metastatic prostate cancer can take years. Broken bones that require surgery to pin and stabilize: liver problems from cancer inside causing blood problems; and pain—the pain that metastatic cancer of the prostate causes to a patient—can only be described as a type of slow torture. Yes, this is a grim reality, so take care of your body, and avoid this happening to you.

18

MALIGNANT MELANOMA

When you look at a mole, you see a large grouping of melanocytes. Larger numbers of melanocytes in close proximity to other melanocytes give a greater risk of one of those cells going kaput. When a melanocyte becomes a melanoma cell, it spreads locally in the mole or nearby skin. A melanoma reaches a certain mass before it is noticeable. Going unnoticed, a melanoma will spread into the lymphatic and blood system, causing doom. (At least one study supports this hypothesis by not disproving it.[113])

Melanoma is on the rise. Currently, your risk is one in fifty-nine.[114]

Most of the advice for skin lesions is to "watch and see if it changes." When you look at the details of this advice, you find a policy of ABCDE for evaluation of skin lesions: asymmetry, border irregularity, color, diameter, and evolution are a good place to start, but they are neither comprehensive nor 100 percent accurate. Cancers are found in lesions that do not flag any of the ABCDE criteria. Some malignant melanoma might even be pink in color (amelanotic) rather than dark. As an individual, you might want to consider that trading a small scar for a skin lesion could be a good option. (If you don't like scars, then accept that you are somewhere between one and fifty-nine in line for malignant melanoma.)

Malignant Melanoma Development.

The development of melanoma is related to the number of melanocytes in a section of skin. Pigmented lesions contain more melanocytes. The more melanocytes in a lesion the higher the risk of melanoma as related to that lesion.

Allen J. Orehek, M.D.

Remember some types of melanoma have no pigment at all - these are very difficult to discover early. Using the ABCDE pattern of recognizing dangerous lesions can help you.

In writing this chapter, I struggled a bit to find a direct answer to your question, "Does this skin lesion need to be removed?" (I know you were asking that!) Well, if you follow my hypothesis, removing a chunk of melanocytes reduces your chance that any of those thousands of cells could become a melanoma.

You need to balance your life between a small scar and an acceptable risk of melanoma. Waiting for a skin lesion to change into what looks like a malignant melanoma (suspicious lesion) has allowed the horse to leave the barn. Consider a balance: if you have a number of skin lesions, get a few of them removed and see what the results are. Entire books have been published on the subjects of "dysplastic nevus" and skin lesions. There are no current agreements in even the simple basic terminology that affects the results.

A biopsy of the lesion is the only way to be sure of what comprises a skin lesion. The diagnosis of skin lesions is a histological one because it is impossible to look with the eye alone to try to tell someone not to worry about it. Some of the lumps and bumps in the skin have a better chance of being identified by your health care team as benign. Other lumps and bumps can be mired down in a bog of guessing what those tiny cells are up to. This chapter is not about all types of skin cancer and skin-related problems. The core is concentration on malignant melanoma. If you have a skin lesion in a cosmetically sensitive location, then punch a chunk out of the worst part of it and identify the cells. If your skin lesion is in a noncosmetic location, then have it removed. I realize that many who read this work may have obstacles in preventing their malignant melanoma, which is why it now affects one in fifty-nine people. Being aware that you have a skin lesion that should be removed is a much different mindset from "watch and wait." You are now empowered with your own personal and unique care of your skin. You now understand the road map of how to be sure you do not develop malignant melanoma that spreads. However, the road ahead may be bumpy.

When the USPSTF set up guidelines on skin cancer in 2008, I was outraged. The guidelines were distant from both my own clinical experience and sheer common sense. In 2008 I started counting cases, and when I got to my eighth melanoma biopsy for the year, I asked a question of a local large dermatology group. The group sees about twelve melanoma cases a year. How is it that a large dermatology practice gets twelve melanoma cases and I picked up eight?[xlvi] The reason is that not all melanoma is by the book. Not all of them appear exactly as a metastatic melanoma looks. I am sure that when a skin lesion looks horrible, then a biopsy might provide the information that it is a cancer. Yet in the earliest stages, the skin lesions could be simply removed, as the biopsy makes the diagnosis. Biopsy of an abnormal skin lesion is the least expensive test that makes the diagnosis.

In my practice I often find skin lesions that are located in critical parts of the body, ones that do not allow much skin to be removed. Rather than ignore them, I do a small biopsy of the area—get the tissue, and find out what the lesion is. Then everyone involved knows whether to observe this skin lesion or excise it. Mohs surgeons are your best friends.[xlvii] You should let only them remove your biopsy-proven skin cancers. Other surgeons will guess that they got all of the cancer by taking a wide sweep around the edge. However, you can be sure only once it is evaluated under a microscope.

Most malignant melanoma will be in Stage III when it is diagnosed. Stage III means that the melanoma cancer has spread to the local lymph tissue in the skin. This is bad. But often people are still cured. The stage of melanoma at the time of diagnosis is important: Stage 0—melanoma in situ; Stage I—located in top layer of skin; Stage II—where there is deeper growth of the

---

xlvi   All eight cases were treated by specialty consultation (Mohs surgeon and plastic surgeons) with wider excision. Some had lymph node biopsy. None had metastatic and all were cured of their cancer.

xlvii   A type of microscopically controlled surgery developed by Frederic Mohs, MD, offering a way to completely remove skin cancer and offer a high cure rate.

melanoma. Removing skin lesions when the melanoma is Stage 0, I, or II will gain the you a significant advantage over removal at a higher stage. Removal of the pigmented lesions before you have developed Stage 0 disease is even a better option. You can prevent malignant melanoma—just keep a close eye on your skin.

19

USPSTF, WTF?

I was able to locate a few different explanations of what the USPSTF is: "The <u>U.S. Preventive Services Task Force</u> was convened by the Public Health Service to rigorously evaluate clinical research in order to assess the merits of preventive measures, including screening tests, counseling, immunizations, and preventive medications." And the USPSTF is "an independent panel of experts in primary care and prevention that systematically reviews the evidence of effectiveness and develops recommendations for clinical preventive services."[115] The task force, a panel of primary care physicians and epidemiologists, is funded, staffed, and appointed by the U.S. Department of Health and Human Services Agency for Healthcare Research and Quality. Both descriptions of what the USPSTF is set up and designed to do makes one believe that it is at the front of the prevention train. This is just not the current situation. I briefly reviewed this idea in the chapter "What This Book Is About," and now I will lay it all at your feet for you to understand some critical points.

You need to realize how you are not given the choice or chance of prevention. If it were the case that your health care provided you the right information about what services you should be getting but the insurance companies did not cover them, that would be one thing. However, the advice you currently get from your health care team is based on USPSTF guidelines. (Many people do not even get that level of care, and that is an extremely sad situation.) Guidelines drive board questions. So your health care team is being trained to follow guideline recommendations. You can see how this can quickly change your medical care into health care.[xlviii]

My view is that you should simply know the truth. A decade from now we will look back in horror at what the USPSTF was doing to the general population. The USPSTF describes itself as an independent panel of private-sector experts. It goes on to state that it is composed of experts in prevention and primary care, who offer the "highest quality clinical preventive services."

I had an initial desire to take the current USPSTF document line by line and provide for you my thoughts on each recommendation that it gave; however, the document is too long (292 pages) to integrate into this writing. [116] I have elected to summarize its deficiencies and give enough attention to its poor overall philosophy that you will understand the need to question what the task force has published. I understand that once you question what the USPSTF has put on the table for 2011, you will then question what advice your health care team is giving you. I hope you will then further question all that the healthcare community has put in front of you.

The length of the document makes it especially difficult for even a dedicated physician to understand what the task force is trying to recommend. A dedicated physician must not only read the document but also read and check the references to

---

xlviii   Medical care based on the art and science of medicine. Health care based on the current system.

see how the authors reached their conclusions. Often the new guidelines prove to be untested. They are often based on data/ studies that are narrow and dubiously applicable.

The USPSTF made broad, sweeping statements that often changed patterns of patient care that had been established for years.[117] A simple review of the 2009 text[118] will be at significant odds with the 2011 recommendations for testicular cancer prevention. In 2008 the USPSTF told people over age seventy-five not to check for colon cancer.[119] Its words were, "Do not screen routinely" for ages seventy-six through eighty-five, and for people over eighty-five, it used the words, "Do not screen." How sad this is when many articles point to the fact that most colon cancer strikes people who never got a colonoscopy and people who in advanced age.[120] I imagine that few members of the USPSTF have sat bedside by a seventy-seven-year-old patient who is puking stool because of a total obstruction from a colon mass. But I also imagine they would understand that without checking and treating the precancer state, this leaves no hope at all for any other options. Worse, the USPSTF totally ignores the fact that when an eighty-two-year-old woman starts to poop blood and cry out in abdominal pain, she will be evaluated for the tumor in her colon.

New guidelines usually were applied to a specific disease state along with a statement explaining that there were not enough data to make a comment. Making a statement that there isn't enough information to make a statement seems hypocritical. Most reasonable people believe that when there are not enough data on a given subject to make a statement, one would make no statement. This is not the case in the works of the USPSTF, as it made a variety of guideline recommendations in situations for which no information was available. You deserve better than this when it comes to your body.

Over a decade of giving detailed care to patients has shown me that age is not important once you reach sixty. Most of my patients can opt out of statistics once they reach age sixty. When it comes to general health and their unique situation, statistics matter less. One who is age sixty living in the United States has an average of twenty-two and a half years remaining. One who is age sixty and has given her body time and attention to prevention is doing very well. Many guidelines use mortality data as an endpoint. If you were to work in a shop and use a metal grinder and not wear proper eye protection, there would be no affect on your mortality. However, you might end up blind from metal entering your eye. When you receive medical advice that is based upon mortality statistics, you need to move past the idea of dying and try to understand more about your quality of life.

In its section on breast cancer, the USPSTF stated that women have a shortened life span once they hit age seventy-five. At age seventy-five, your life expectancy is still twelve years. I do not interpret that data to suggest that your life span is shortened. When you are seventy-six, the best way to make seventy-seven is to take care of yourself.

Now it gets a bit ugly to follow along, mostly because this is a bit complicated (and pretty revolting—sorry). But this is what the USPSTF has thrown down. Because of how knotty the guidelines are, with different grades to their recommendations and statements, it's difficult to summarize any specific disease process. For instance, with regards to breast cancer, the USPSTF recommended screening with mammography every two years from age fifty through seventy-four and stopping after age seventy-five. Don't do self-exams.[121] The word *"insufficient"* appears in the sections that relate to MRI of breast and to women of age forty. The authors admitted that old age is the most important risk factor for breast cancer in women, yet the task force recommended that women stop doing any evaluation at age seventy-four. How could the USPSTF authors recommend against screening the population they admitted faces the highest risk? If you are seventy-five, you should be outraged. (An important side note is that the breasts in women under age fifty are usually fibrous, and the fibrous tissue can limit the usefulness of the mammogram. So if a manual exam detects something suspicious but your mammogram is negative, you should continue evaluating. You are unique, and there is no way that as a woman in her forties you want to ignore a lump.) The USPSTF went on to explain that "in recent decades, the early detection of breast cancer has been accomplished by physical examination by a clinician (CBE), by a woman herself (BSE), or by mammography." Yet its final recommendation was apparently blind to this fact.

The USPSTF based its data on a study called Canadian National Breast Screening Study–2: 13-year results of a randomized trial in women aged 50–59. The data appear based upon a question asked by NIH.[122] As the basic question and subsequent data may not apply to you, then how did the USPSTF make a sweeping recommendation to include age groups that were not studied?

My own evaluation is correct and is based primarily on a Canadian study that was completed in 2000.[123] This study showed that when adding mammogram to breast exam alone, there was no significant difference in mortality. Review of these data could indicate that in 1985 the Canadian authors knew that doing a breast self-exam would be beneficial. The conclusion of the study for women aged fifty to fifty-nine years stated that the addition of annual mammography screening to physical examination had no impact on breast cancer mortality. Realize that when this study was completed, digital mammography was not available—a repeat of this study now would have *much* different results. The pain in all of this is that what the USPSTF gave as a final recommendation was not what was designed and studied.

The USPSTF mentioned the "preventable burden, potential harms, costs, and current practice" of the breast exam, but there was absolutely no paragraph or heading listing the benefits.[124] Seriously, how do you expect a woman to hurt herself by doing a breast self-examination? This section further detailed that the USPSTF's concern was "anxiety and breast cancer worry, as well as repeated visits and unwarranted imaging and biopsies." If you want to prevent a cancer, you have to work hard. There is simply no easy ride when it comes to understanding all of the factors that can go wrong or right when it comes to your breasts. Men reading this are not out of the spotlight either. Male breast cancer affects two thousand men a year.[xlix] Woman or man, please check your breasts once a month. If you find a lump, contact a physician who understands that the next step is to prevent the burdens of unneeded radiation, unnecessary surgery, and excessive stress. In the next decade, we will discover the harm that the USPSTF injected into the community by recommending against doing a breast self-examination. We will see a time when all people simply check their breasts and get an idea of any new lumps or bumps.

As the USPSTF discussed the use of digital mammography, its concern was that although "overall detection is somewhat higher with digital mammography ... [it] is not clear whether this additional detection would lead to reduced mortality from breast cancer." [125] Well, let me make it clear to you: detecting the cancer before it spreads allows the patient to live longer. We need no study for that thought process. It is simply common sense. If there is an institution with money to blow, then I ask it to please study mortality in a population who has a cancer detected before it spreads compared to a population who has a cancer that has already spread. I am confident that the results will show that when people detect and treat a cancer before it spreads, they generally do better than those treated for a metastatic cancer.

---

xlix   The American Cancer Society estimates that about two thousand new cases of invasive breast cancer are diagnosed in men each year and approximately four hundred fifty men die from breast cancer annually.

The USPSTF said the same thing about magnetic resonance imaging (MRI). More cases of cancer are detected with mammography, but somehow it "is unknown whether detecting these additional cases of cancer would lead to reduced breast cancer mortality."[126] Well, it is unknown because it has not been studied. The USPSTF should have applied some common sense here and realized that detecting a cancer early is always better than detecting it late. It suggested that MRI yields more false-positive results than a mammogram does. My response is that the doctors reading the MRI need to understand what they are doing. Powerful technology in the hands of physicians who are not properly trained yields poor results.

Sometimes as I read the recommendations from a preventive task force, I recall the classic stop-motion Christmas television special *Rudolph the Red-Nosed Reindeer*.[127] On the Island of Misfit Toys, we meet a jack-in-the-box named Charlie, a toy train with square wheels, and a boat that doesn't float. As I read recommendations from a preventive task force that doesn't actually advocate for prevention, I often envision the Island of Misfit Toys as a good place for its central office.

Here are some of the summary statements that reflect the strategy of "don't look, don't tell, don't find it, wait for it to become a problem first," which lies on the other side of the fence from real prevention.

SCREENING FOR SKIN CANCER: "Insufficient [data] to balance harms and benefits." I like this statement better than saying "don't do it at all"; at least here we understand that it is a subject that has not been directly studied. Common sense tells you that when you look at the skin, you might notice more than if you do not look at the skin. (I have more details in the section on melanoma and skin.)

SCREENING FOR ABDOMINAL AORTIC ANEURYSM: Smokers over age sixty-five get a one-time screen. Other than that, no one else gets a thumbs-up to go get checked. Yet AAA kills fifteen thousand people and disables even more.[128] It should also be noted that the USPSTF recommendation set one hundred cigarettes as the defining criteria for being a smoker. Yet no one has looked at secondhand smoke—how does living or working in that environment affect a person? Before many places banned smoking indoors, everyone who worked in such a place would have been exposed to significant doses for years. If you are a retired worker from Dunkin' Donuts before it went smoke free, you might have had exposure to more than one hundred cigarettes. Consider getting checked.

SCREENING FOR CAROTID ARTERY STENOSIS: The task force recommended against screening for asymptomatic carotid artery stenosis in general adult population.[i] As I have discussed in detail previously in this work, why would you wait for a stroke to tell you that you have a big problem? We never hear a health care provider telling you to "wait for your diabetes to cause some symptoms before you treat it," or "wait for your hypertension to cause a symptom before you treat it." So why would you not treat something that is so critical to your well-being and quality of life?

SCREENING FOR CHRONIC OBSTRUCTIVE PULMONARY DISEASE USING SPIROMETRY: The task force recommended against it. If it remained true to its definition of a smoker—one hundred cigarettes, which would include scores of secondhand smokers— then again you have a huge population who might benefit. The cost of COPD is estimated to be $800 billion over the next twenty years.[129] Evaluation with spirometry is simple and costs Medicare about $35 one time. The task force did state that if you are over age fifty, you need to get your annual flu shot. Every day, wherever we look, the flu shot is pushed and advertised with an annual price tag, not a one-time cost. One really must try to comprehend who wrote the guidelines. Health care will go on ignoring evaluation of an asymptomatic problem in

---

i   Screening for carotid artery stenosis part of the USPTDF 2011 document.

prior tobacco users. However, medical attention to this problem is possible for you if you simply look out for your own needs. You are the captain of your own ship—it is up to you to set your destination. I am happy to work as a master gunner on your ship for you!

SCREENING FOR COLORECTAL CANCER: USPSTF recommended screening for colorectal cancer using fecal occult blood testing, sigmoidoscopy, or colonoscopy in adults, beginning at age fifty and continuing until age seventy-five.[130] Doing fecal cards is better than nothing at all, and doing a sigmoidoscopy might help if your polyp or cancer is toward the end of the colon, but a colonoscopy is the best way to make sure your colon is free from polyps. When it comes to ages seventy-six through eighty-five, the USPSTF recommended against routine screening for colorectal cancer in adults. This statement is a general, sweeping statement about age rather than about prevention of a disease. The USPSTF did state that there might be considerations that support colorectal cancer screening in an individual patient. It is not clear to me why one would stop treating a patient at age eighty-five when an individual still has six and a half years left, on average. I totally disagree with giving up on a patient. A ninety-year-old who has taken care of his body has no competing causes of mortality that outweigh any harm. As the guidelines start at age fifty, who is to hold the hand of all the poor buggers who were not even fifty and developed colon or rectal cancer. A thirty-eight year old who received information from the **MPC** was floored when a dime-sized polyp was removed from his colon. No one would debate that as an individual he would have been dealing with a diagnosis of colon cancer before he was even forty-five. A colon prep and a missed day of work will be worth their weight in gold for him for the rest of his life—dodging the bullet of colon cancer is something to celebrate.

Many published medical articles have discussed and reviewed ways to prevent colon cancer, and most of the published data agree that removing precancerous polyps from the colon prevent colon cancer. Once you consider that getting your colon checked decreases your chance of getting colon cancer, you have no need to go any further. Get into the hands of a GI specialist who does colonoscopies all day long, and get your colonoscopy. If you have no other reason, once you are a few decades old-get one every few years. There is more information on this topic in the colon cancer prevention section.

SCREENING FOR OVARIAN CANCER: "The U.S. Preventive Services Task Force (USPSTF) recommends against routine screening for ovarian cancer."[131] This is hard to comprehend, given that ovarian cancer kills and harms about forty thousand women a year.[132] It is the ninth most common cancer in women. Once it is discovered, mortality is very high. Most women get chemotherapy and perhaps an operation (sounds expensive!). All that was needed to prevent this painful expensive mess was for a woman to know what her ovaries were doing. The CA–125 test might be helpful once you have the disease. But many tissues and noncancer problems can produce CA–125, so this test is not independently conclusive. The USPSTF said, "Because there is a low incidence of ovarian cancer in the general population (age-adjusted incidence of 17 per 100,000 women), screening for ovarian cancer is likely to have a relatively low yield. The great majority of women with a positive screening test will not have ovarian cancer."[133] I do not believe that any woman who is suffering with ovarian cancer will find any consolation in this final statement.

SCREENING FOR PROSTATE CANCER: The plan for prostate cancer is even more confusing. The USPSTF concluded "that the current evidence is insufficient to assess the balance of benefits and harms of prostate cancer screening in men younger than age 75." The USPSTF also recommended against screening for prostate cancer in men age seventy-five years and older. Again, the task force made my idea simple: it is a preventive task force that gives no helpful advice.

So it happens that just about every one of the USPSTF's recommendations aimed at saving money. It listed nothing that covers you should you have disease. You only get packed into a bunch of people who have a "small" chance of developing the problem.

We can all have our own opinions and follow the path in life that best suits us. If you fail to determine and choose an individual path regarding your health care, you will blindly go to your death with some aspect of a treatable medical condition with the rest of the population you match.[134]

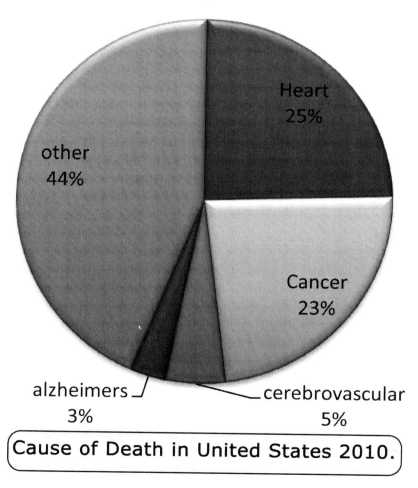

Cause of Death in United States 2010.

John Ritter died from an aortic dissection. He was fifty-four years old. Apparently, this disorder affects about ten thousand people in the United States each year. Many more have the disorder and have no idea that they have it. When the dissection hits, your chance of making it out of the hospital alive is limited.[135] You often hear that some diseases or problems are not preventable. I will challenge those statements time and time again.

I believe the USPSTF was wrong to ignore life expectancy and recommend stopping Medical Prevention at certain ages. Why would one stop an evaluation for cervical, breast, or prostate cancer in the ages that are of the highest risk? If recommendations from a task force had been in place for a number of years and a given disease had been all but eradicated, then decreasing the amount of attention on that disease would make sense. But as long as hundreds of thousands of people in the United States die from preventable diseases, more should be done, not less.

The logo of the USPSTF is the caduceus. This represents the wand of the Greek god Hermes and is often associated with commercial endeavors. I agree that the USPSTF is a commercial endeavor and not a medical organization of prevention. I understand that some of you reading this book have done work for the USPSTF. I urge you to make the following changes:

- Integrate my pain and suffering equation into your work as you evaluate cost.

- Realize the least expensive test is the one that makes the diagnosis.

- Do not despair if not everyone listens to your advice.

- Prepare your own medical studies to verify your results before you pass down a mass guideline.

- And finally, treat humans as unique individuals and not as part of a general population.

When a doctor is in training, she first cuts a worm then a frog then a cat. Then she dissects a cadaver, and then she works on humans. A new drug is first tested chemically then on animal subjects then on a limited number of compensated volunteers, and then the drug is released for general consumption. When the USPSTF released its guidelines, they were untested. (Yes, untested by the USPSTF; it did not put the guidelines to the test before delivering them to your physician's front door). The task force simply made a statement and "hoped like hell" it would work. They have put so much pressure on the corporate bottom line that the care of people has been forsaken. I mentioned previously that doctors are psychologically abandoning the people whom they care for. By not even giving patients the options to reduce their chance of "doom," they are not providing medical care.

The USPSTF often worked with pooled meta-analysis data. The following story illustrates the problem with this approach:

You like soup. Your town has three restaurants that serve soup, so a study is completed. Restaurant A serves soup and has one hundred cars leaving that lot every day. Restaurant B has only forty cars per day, and Restaurant C has only twenty cars per day. So the data would suggest that because people go to Restaurant A more often, it must provide the best soup. If you were a task force, your final thought would be that everyone should go to Restaurant A. You personally may not like the soup there at all, but others do.

You are unique. You cannot be fit into the mass population in every situation. You should never draw a conclusion from a meta-analysis, unless the conclusion is that you need to study the data further. Use the meta-analysis to make decisions about what would be a good topic to study. I would be able to write a study that shows people who leave an orthopedic office tend to have more casts than ones who leave the eye doctor. And the ones who leave the eye doctor seem to have more problems being able to drive. So it must be that eye doctors aren't good for the eye. And if you go to an orthopedic doctor, there is a good chance that you will need a cane or a cast or a brace. So will you decide it's best not to go to the orthopedist? Or will you decide that people who go to the orthopedic specialist need treatments that result in casts? So you can pick where you want to go for your soup, and you may try all three places, but if they don't make it the way you want it, you will not go back. (Note: None of the studies ever even checked to see how often someone had hair in his or her soup!) Do not rely on anything that is given to you as a meta-analysis. I can take any 110 studies and then select 30 of them on a subject to come up with whatever results I want.

Rather than dumping down the care that is provided to all patients, what is needed is allowing them access to physicians who understand the issues—the anxiety of discovery, the chances of an unnecessary test, the possibility of false-negative and genuine false-positive test results, and coordination with a good surgical team for biopsy and possibly excision. Physicians need to understand good pathology and have a good team of oncology specialists who understand current treatments. Doctors are bright people—why not push what they can do a bit?

20

WHAT CAN I DO TO HELP MYSELF?

Your best advice will come from a physician you trust. Often people move, and many physicians move or stop practicing. People end up going to large practices with nurse practitioners and physician assistants. Remember some nurse practitioners and certified physician assistants are better than physicians, as they could be more likely to simply say, "I don't know what that is—Here is a referral." I want everyone to know that I say those words every single day—we can't know it all!

If your doctor blindly follows national guidelines (which in some cases provide the basis of board certifications), then your care could be in danger. If your doctor ignores guidelines altogether, you should be even more worried. If you have a health care provider who looks at the guidelines, discusses them with you, and then applies a plan understanding that you are unique, then you are in good shape.

When you go for a pap smear and you are told "No news is good news," just chuckle and ask to send you the results. In my office I tell people, "Nothing means nothing." We call with the results. So when your health care provider tells you that no news is good news, you should hear, "We are too lazy and disorganized to call you with your results"—or even worse, "We don't really care enough about you to be sure to let you know the results." Sadly, for a few patients, I have requested old records that revealed an abnormal pap smear the patient never knew about. Be sure you have good communication with your health care providers and a full understanding of the results of testing that you have already completed.

I am often asked about the value of whole body scans. They may be instructive. For the most part, I use radiology with radiation only to confirm some earlier finding or suspicion. Used in that way, it is very sensitive. Scanning the whole body needs to be done without putting you at risk of more radiation. Some locations might offer you a multiple-hour full MRI scan—this is a good start. If you are going to have each part of your body evaluated by MRI, and if that data meet the standards of the **MPC**, then you have spent time wisely. Scanning the entire body is only part of what you need to be doing. Prevention of dementia requires many other details that scans and images cannot provide for you. Many cancers will not be prevented by whole body scans—you need scopes. Evaluation of the heart valves will be missed on a whole body scan—you need a 2-D echo. Other important details are also missed by only a whole body scan, so stay organized—do your homework. While working on the final revision of this book, I discovered a place called the Medical Prevention Center of Hamburg , and it seems that it is well on its way toward offering Medical Prevention in its own style.

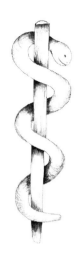

DEMENTIA PREVENTION CENTER™

2637 E ATLANTIC BLVD #19129
PAMPANO BEACH, FLORIDA 33062
www.dementiapreventioncenter.com | info@dementiapreventioncenter.com
www.medicalpreventioncenter.com | info@medicalpreventioncenter.com

Feburary 21, 2012

President Barack Obama
The White House
1600 Pennsylvania Avenue NW
Washington, DC 20500

Dear President Obama,

RE: The prevention of dementia is possible.

The details are in the book Prevention is Difficult awaiting publication. I have put thousands of hours of work and research into this project. Over a decade of studying medicine, treating people, curing disease, learning by errors, and understanding the system has come together to illuminate what one needs to do in the prevention of Alzheimer's disease. (I am not boasting that I am the best physician, as I know many that are smarter and brighter. Nonetheless, I can hold my own).

One will not find what I am teaching coming from any of the expert review boards or a committee. "The Micron Stroke Hypothesis of Alzheimer's Disease and Dementia, " accepted for publication by *Journal of Medical Hypothesis* on January 9, 2012 (doi:10.1016/j.mehy.2012.01.020). A new medical term is introduced, **Micron Stroke**.

Every fifty-year-old male who has a history of major tobacco use has carotid artery stenosis of some degree. I can only hope the report wasn't "no significant carotid artery stenosis," as the true risk and damage being done will not be known for years.

Sincerely,

Allen J. Orehek, M.D

MEDICAL PREVENTION CENTER™

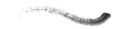

It wasn't until this work was well underway, specifically as I wrote early versions of the chapters on thyroid cancer and Alzheimer's disease, that I realized many people reading this book will have additional questions. Some will need additional direction or will be interested in further Medical Prevention. This work is not intended to be a long-winded advertisement for the **MEDICAL PREVENTION CENTER**.— But as it progressed, it was clear that unique individuals who want additional help could have a difficult time in getting the help they desire. I established **MPC** so if you are a motivated individual you can visit us online. (www.medicalpreventioncenter.com). You will be asked questions like "How big are the blockages in your neck?" "What is the size of your left atrium?" "When was the last scope to your stomach?" "Do your kidneys have any masses on them?" This is an uncommon approach to health care. This is a controversial approach to your medical needs. You will be stimulated into correctly understanding your body. If you are well informed, then you will have a better idea what questions you should ask when you see a health care provider about your medical problems. Your current pathway of Medical Prevention does not provide many of the approaches covered in this book because current guidelines do not cover this science. The information from the **MPC** is not based upon what your insurance company says you can and cannot do—that is your health care. The "homework" is not based on current guidelines primarily concerned about specific resources—that is your health care. Your work will be in understanding the condition of your body—medicine. This is where you get specific data based on current technology and trends, avoid invasive procedures and unnecessary testing, and use only the medications needed and at the lowest dose necessary for the shortest period.[li] You still need a health care team to help you reach your goals. I am a doctor, but I am not *your* doctor!

You can set a goal of completing prevention in all sixteen categories. You will get a feather for your cap for sure. You would then prevent many of the diseases that you observe in those around you as you age. The **MPC** is also a valuable resource for people you love and might be concerned about. I often ask myself how it is that a family gets involved with Mom or Dad

---

li   You will still need your own personal health care team. **MPC** provides only extremely detailed information.

only when the dementia reaches a moderate and problematic level. Why were these people not given the ability to undergo a simple $150 test to make the specific discoveries and then be able to prevent those diseases a decade ago? Prevention with the coordinated and organized effort of the **MPC** costs less than the first month of an active disease. The coordinated plan to prevent dementia from the **DEMENTIA PREVENTION CENTER** costs less than the first few months spent in a personal care or dementia center. If you are interested, you have options to have us review your data and give them specific comments and scores. The information from **MPC** Certified study utilizes medical teams that detail what they see and report important details that may also serve as your baseline for future evaluations. **MPC** Certified teams performing the tests do so with unparalleled quality, partly because the specific requirements and prerequisites for a completed test are thorough and detailed. Testing and reports can be completed anyplace in the world and forwarded for review and comments. When a completed test has the **MPC** Certified stamp, you will know that report was evaluated and found to be acceptable. If your data are superficial or the health care team did not complete your evaluation, you will have tools to get started—such as comments about where your health care team went wrong. The details of your organs need to be evaluated, and you can gather that data at many places across the world. Once you have that information, you will be on your way to preventing pain and suffering. We work best when the provider of your service is on board with giving you a **MPC** Certified study—generally you will face a small battle trying to get quality information with the proper details. Yes, a perfect example of how prevention is difficult. Always get medical recommendations from your health care team, as we can provide you only information, not advice.

Those of you who really enjoy challenging things in life may decide to visit the **DEMENTIA PREVENTION CENTER**. Here you will be engaged into a comprehensive thought process that few can complete without unique discoveries. The discoveries can prevent your dementia—or work to mitigate worsening of your dementia if you are already on your way down that path.

I understand that many of you after reading this book will put in the significant amount of time necessary for true prevention. You will celebrate preventing the significant amount of pain and suffering that was otherwise awaiting you. Some of you may have followed other preventive approaches and were misled. Perhaps you were even hurt from incorrect diagnoses, wrong tests, or complications. I wish you were my direct patient and I were able to provide to you the detailed care that you deserve.

The **MPC** does not have patients. You will have your own health care or medical team. This allows us to give full and detailed explanations of your specific and unique needs based upon any information you provide to us. Medicalpreventioncenter.com will provide you the tools that you need to be successful in preventing disease. Getting a completion certificate from the **MPC** will earn you not only the glory but also the satisfaction of knowing that you have done your part to take care of the machine that you are. Perhaps even someday—get you a discount on your life or long-term care insurance.

Over the next few decades, advances in technology will help us visualize the inner workings of the body even more. We might not know the exact process of some disease states at this time, but establishing the foundation for how to use forthcoming information will be important to improving the quality of life of those around us. Obtaining additional technology and treatments in the future will only be as good as having a thorough method of applying them. As I explained in detail about the *micron stroke*, an entire world exists at the level of the nano stroke, the destruction of a single neuron-to-neuron connection in the brain. Well out of reach of our current scientific technology to understand, it is a concept that deserves attention. Once medicine and science start to consider new concepts—the rate of original discoveries and treatments will explode. The cure for many problems is not in doing more of the same that has been done—rather in doing things a bit different.

While I was gathering the material for this book, I met with a number of scientists and physicians, all at different stages in their careers. More often than not, they were intrigued by the content and design of my Medical Prevention plan. Many of them wanted to adopt some of this new philosophy into their own practice treatment plans. Unfortunately, their employers and the insurance industry restrict them. I cannot do much to change that, but what I can change is the understanding and intent of people like you. Many doctors who are restricted to providing health care would love to again become a physician of medicine—their hearts yearn for it. Evaluate your health care team carefully, I am certain that many of you will still find physicians of medicine who, while sticking close to the health care agenda, are taking good care of your medical needs. Many physicians are incredibly dedicated and dynamic people. Feel free to push them a little bit—they work great under pressure.

Not everything in this book can be applied to everyone. I can teach many people to shave without cutting themselves, and yet some of them still will. When you apply my recommendations for prevention, you need to approach them as a unique individual with your own unique needs.

21

WHAT ELSE CAN BE DONE?

One might not think much of this effort I have put forth if I were not able to offer some insight to the current problems facing our country. Well, I have given the current health care system the same thought and attention I have given the specific diseases I have written about. I hope the concepts in *The Micron Stroke Hypothesis of Alzheimer's Disease and Dementia* lead to new discoveries across the world. In a decade, the way that we evaluate something such as dementia will be a direct about-face from what is done today.

In 2010 Medicare spent about $523 billion, and this massive spending is sometimes called the "Medicare Crisis."[136] A concerted effort by the people of the United States could solve this crisis. First, you can understand that it is not so much a crisis as it is a discrepancy of where the payment for services goes.

The current Medicare system operates by assigning a reimbursement cost to a service. Medicare covers 80 percent of a fee; 20 percent is left either to the individual or to secondary insurance.

Someone without any medical insurance could go to an emergency room and end up with a bill for $2500. Medicare's rate on the same service could be $147.90 (dozens of current procedural terminology codes fit this situation), and the person who has Medicare would be responsible for 20 percent of that amount.

We can develop a new system. This system—call it "Mediunited"—could be started with a separate policy or law. The law will cover those without Medicare. What the law will encompass is not an 80/20 system but rather a 20/80 system. The individual will pay for Mediunited on a monthly basis. The covered individual will have a Mediunited card and access to medical care. When the person goes for medical attention or treatment, he will be responsible for 80 percent of the Medicare-approved rate for that service. In the example where the Medicare rate was $147.90, Mediunited will pay 20 percent and the individual will pay 80 percent. The individual could seek a private insurance plan (from a free and open market) to cover that 80 percent. But with the current cost of insurance premiums, many individuals would be well ahead in the financial books by paying the 80 percent themselves. For the Mediunited plan to work, it will need to be set up like Medicare, as a federal organization. Laws would have to ensure there were no significant restriction in care and no prior authorizations. There will not be any of the administrative hassles that are commonly found in private health insurance plans. The plan will work extremely well for people who remain healthy. The plan should be made available for a low cost. The plan's monthly fee should be adjusted each year to cover the expenses of the prior year. By pooling all of the covered people together, it is possible that the rate could be adjusted much lower. Part of the law that gives birth to Mediunited should stipulate that when funds put into the kitty greatly exceed the amount of outgoing payments, then money is used to reduce the following year's fee or is refunded as a lower premium.

Blanketing the entire United States with this plan will be best after a few years of test running in a study population. Those excluded from Mediunited will be those who already receive help from welfare, medical assistance, or public programs. Those who qualify for Medicare will not participate in Mediunited. Even those who are not legal citizens could participate in this plan. Actuarial teams will be responsible for keeping track of the funds in and funds out. For those who had a Mediunited card, the more they consume, the more for which they are responsible. To fully map out a plan like this and address all the inevitable counterarguments would take pages beyond measure. But I hope this gives you an idea.

People speak of the medically uninsured and how they place a burden on the health system. We could make "uninsured" an official, card-carrying status. A person meeting certain criteria (similar to a driver's license—somewhat selective but widely accessible) could get an "uninsured card." With this card people could get medical attention wherever they usually go—the emergency room, the office, the clinic. They will pay no bill, and the facility providing the service will get a tax credit/refund based on the Medicare-approved rate for the service provided. This would allow the uninsured of America to have the burden placed across the entire United States. No longer will a location of economic downturn doom a local hospital. All of America will join in taking care of their brothers and sisters who are down on their luck. Perhaps it will not be the most popular method of payment in doctors' offices and hospitals. But as a private physician, I will not have to go far to form a network of other doctors who see and treat such people under those terms. Being able to provide care and get a break on taxes would be a tremendous help to all involved.

The subtle difference here is that when someone who is providing health care pays taxes, she generates income and jobs for many others also. This is night and day compared to Medicare, where the government foots the bill. If one is able to understand how the finances are different in the two situations, then please speak with me more on this subject and see if we can help out our brothers and sisters who have no medical insurance and nowhere to turn.

GRAB A PEN: On the first calendar,

AUGUST '20--						
S	M	T	W	Th	F	S
1	2	3	4	5	6	7
8	9	10	11	12	13	14
15	16	17	18	19	20	21
22	23	24	25	26	27	28
29	30	31				

SEPTEMBER '20--						
S	M	T	W	Th	F	S
				1	2	3	4
5	6	7	8	9	10	11
12	13	14	15	16	17	18
19	20	21	22	23	24	25
26	27	28	29	30		

OCTOBER '20--						
S	M	T	W	Th	F	S
3	4	5	6	7	8	
10	11	12	13	14	15	16
17	18	19	20	21	22	23
24	25	26	27	28	29	30
31						

- went to doctor got BP checked

NOVEMBER '20--						
S	M	T	W	Th	F	S
21	22	23	24	25	26	27
28	29	30				

DECEMBER '20-						
S	M	T	W	Th	F	S
			1	2	3	4
5	6	7	8	9	10	
12	13	14	15			
19	20	21	22	23	24	25
26	27	28	29	30	31	

- had labs done and visit with doctor

JANUARY '20--						
S	M	T	W	Th	F	S
						1
23	24	25	26	27	28	29
30	31					

FEBRUARY '20--						
S	M	T	W	Th	F	S
		1	2	3	4	5
6	7	8	9	10	11	12
13	14	15	16	17	18	19
20	21	22	23	24	25	26
27	28					

MARCH '20--						
S	M	T	W	Th	F	S
		1	2	3		
6	7	8	9	10	11	12
13	14					
20	21					
27	28	29	30	31		

had check up 'everything ok

APRIL '20--						
S	M	T	W	Th	F	S
					1	2
3	4	5	6	7	8	9
10	11	12	13	14	15	
17	18	19	20	21	22	23
24	25	26	27	28	29	30

MAY '20--						
S	M	T	W	Th	F	S
1	2	3	4	5	6	7
29	30	31				

- Flu shot at the pharmacy

JUNE '20--						
S	M	T	W	Th	F	S
			1	2	3	4
5	6	7	8	9	10	11
12	13	14	15	16	17	18
19	20	21	22	23	24	25
26	27	28	29	30		

JULY '20--						
S	M	T	W	Th	F	S
					1	2
3	4	5	6	7	8	9
10	11	12	13	14	15	16
17	18	19	20	21	22	23
24	25	26	27	28	29	30
31						

make a circle on the dates that you have actually been to the doctor in the last year. Next, fill in the circle on any dates of your medical visits where you worked on prevention. It's quite possible that you have marked a few visits over the year, but you were unable to fill in any circles indicating that you did any disease prevention. If you are a lucky person and did fill in a circle because of prevention, next, write the organ or disease process that you worked on for prevention (using a female as example here). Not many people reading this work have matched the list on the next page.

If your calendar has no filled-in boxes, and if you did not come close to matching the prevention list, the fact is simply you are not preventing any of these diseases. Now look at the disease problems listed in the box. How many medical visits do you think will be spent in treating any one of those problems? How many medical visits will occur in just the first two months after a serious diagnosis of one of those problems?

Remember to count consultations with specialists, biopsy results, chemotherapy, radiation therapy, follow-up, and anything else related. The individual who discovers he has developed that medical situation will have many visits. Likely, the patient would love it if that weren't necessary.

AUGUST '20--

S	M	T	W	Th		
1	2	3	4	5		
8	9	10	11	12		
15	16	17	18	19		
22	23	24	25	26		
29	30	31				

SEPTEMBER '20--

11 assignments.
consult with GI for EGD and Colonoscopy
EGD day
Colonoscopy day
2D echo
Carotid artery ultrasound AAA evaluation
Abdominal ultrasound studies
Thyroid ultrasound
Skin clinic -
                excision f/u
Breast exam and Pelvic
Mammogram

OCTOBER '20--

S	M	T	W	Th		
3	4	5	6	7		
10	11	12	13	⊘		
17	18	19	20	21		
24	25	26	27	28		
31						

DECEMBER '20--

S	M	T	W	Th	F	S
			1	2	3	4
5	6	7	8	9	10	11
12	13	14	15	16	17	18
19	20	21	22	23	24	25
26	27	28	29	30	31	

JANUARY '20--

S	M	T	W	Th	F	S
						1
2	3	4	5	6	7	8
9	10	11	⊘	13	14	15
16	⊘	18	19	20	21	22
23	24	25	26	27	28	29
30	31					

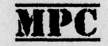

**Sample Schedule
female 5th decade**

FEBRUARY '20--

S	M	T	W	Th	F	S
		1	⊘	3	4	5
6	⊘	8	9	10	11	12
13	14	15	16	17	18	19
20	21	⊘	23	24	25	26
27	28					

MARCH '20--

S	M	T	W	Th	F	S
		1	2	3	4	5
6	7	8	⊘	10	11	12
13	14	15	16	17	⊘	19
20	21	22	23	24	25	26
27	28	29	30	31		

APRIL '20--

S	M	T	W	Th	F	S
					1	2
3	4	⊘	6	7	8	9
10	11	12	13	14	15	16
17	18	19	20	⊘	22	23
24	25	26	27	28	29	30

MAY '20--

S	M	T	W	Th	F	S
1	2	3	4	5	6	7
8	9	10	11	⊘	13	14
15	16	17	18	19	20	21
22	23	24	25	26	27	28
29	30	31				

JUNE '20--

S	M	T	W	Th	F	S
			1	2	3	4
5	6	7	8	9	10	11
12	13	14	15	16	17	18
19	20	21	22	23	24	25
26	27	28	29	30		

JULY '20--

S	M	T	W	Th	F	S
					1	2
3	4	5	6	7	8	9
10	11	12	13	14	15	16
17	18	19	20	21	22	23
24	25	26	27	28	29	30
31						

SUNDAY	MONDAY	TUESDAY	WEDNESDAY	THURSDAY	FRIDAY	SATURDAY
						1 *ER visit for abdominal pain....*
2	3 *Go over CT results with doctor Tim*	4	5	6 *Visit with surgeon for options*	7 *CT of chest today and Labs*	8
9	10	11 *meet with cardiac team for clearance*	12 *Stress test*	13	14 *EKG LABS Chest XRAY*	15
16	17 *meet with chemo team today*	18	19	20	21 *surgery visit today & Dr Tim*	22
23	24	25 *LABS*	26 *Prior auth for PET scan + visit Dr Tim*	27	28	29
30	31					

SUNDAY	MONDAY	TUESDAY	WEDNESDAY	THURSDAY	FRIDAY	SATURDAY
						1
2	3 *PET SCAN*	4 *chemo*	5	6 *Lab day*	7	8
9	10	11 *Chemo*	12	13	14	15
16	17	18	19	20	21	22
23	24	25	26	27	28	29
30	31					

I can easily say that you probably have a number of problems currently active in your body that you are just not aware of. Some of these things can be as common as one in fifty (such as having a bicuspid aortic valve). For some of these things, your body will warn you only when it is already too late. For some, you get no warning at all. You have not done anything specifically related to prevention, and it's not your fault. It is simply the case that no one has ever explained to you what you need to look for in your body. Finding out what exactly is in your body that makes you a unique individual will greatly reduce the pain and suffering in your life. Priorities can be made for people with a family history or a unique situation that stimulates them to further evaluation. There would be some acceptance that a sixty-five-year-old is going to have a higher priority than a forty-one-year-old for colorectal cancer. However, even this simple statement is not always true, as colorectal cancer can occur in some individuals even as teenagers.

I know as you approach the end of the book you might be thinking, "Come on—just tell me what I have to do!" As prevention of dementia by the **DPC** is not a simple set of guidelines or a list that fits everyone, I am going to take you through the example of a sixty-two-year-old female who has completed her **DPC** evaluation. Alessandra was given her "homework" assignment—a book from the **DPC**. Once she read and understood what she needed to do next, she started by making an appointment with her health care team. Alessandra was lucky, as her health care team included a certified physician assistant whom she had known for years—a good working relationship for heath issues. Alessandra had an episode of vision loss last year and was told it was a type of migraine headache. Lately, her memory seems to be less sharp. Before reading *Prevention Is Difficult—But Possible,* she thought it was an expected part of getting older. She was well prepared with the proper handouts from **DPC** for her health care team on the day of her medical visit. Arrangements were made to get the proper testing completed. Although it seemed to stress the patient–doctor relationship because of the amount of time, the rest of it went over perfectly. As the labs were nonfasting, she went there first. Fourteen vials of blood seemed like a lot at first, but when she was done, she felt fine. Over the next three months, she completed a **DPC** Certified MRI of the brain, a carotid artery ultrasound, and a neuropsychological evaluation. Working as the CEO of a steel company, she was always pressed for time; anything extra in her life always needed to sacrifice something else. She reported the data to the **DPC** as she was able to obtain the results. She did have to call the location that did the MRI of her brain and complain about the fact they did not report all of the proper details. But the outpatient MRI center was more than happy to adjust the report after she complained. The neuropsychological evaluation took about six hours over three days—but she found it all very interesting.

When Alessandra had completed the cardiac aspect of her **DPC** testing, she was surprised to discover that her left atrium was of a size that required monitoring for atrial fibrillation to complete her membership score at the **DPC**. Her left atrium was at 52 mm because of severe mitral stenosis. She felt anxious once she re-alized that her mitral valve was pretty much shot—and a valve replacement was in her future. "How did no one ever know that I had this problem?" seemed to play over and over in her mind. "What else can be wrong with me that I do not know about. Is everything going to be okay?" Alessandra faced a day where she had to understand that there were problems with her body that she was not aware of—but she did fine—and ap-proached each condition as if she were dealing with a shipped cancellation from a company that went bankrupt or a truckload of product that was damaged in shipment.

After completing her thirty-day monitor for atrial fibrillation, her health care team told her that she had atrial fibrillation and should start treatment immediately. Many of her other issues seemed to spin around in her head. Her LDL was 58 after four months of treatment with Crestor. She quit tobacco about twenty years earlier but had 20-49 percent stenosis in both carotid arter-ies. The MRI of her brain showed atrophy of the frontal lobes and diffuse white matter changes. She did not pass the neuropsychiatric testing—with a score in the range of moderate cognitive dysfunction. The **DPC** indicated in comments on her membership account that use of medications should be considered to mitigate any further decline in any person with her results. A summer meeting with her health care team resulted in prescriptions for Aricept and Namenda—a visit to a heart surgeon—treatment with Coumadin for her atrial fibrillation—baby aspirin—and, on top of everything else, a referral for a sleep study because she had hypoxia overnight once it was checked for.

Two years later, Alessandra believes her memory is sharper than ever. A small scar under her right breast reminds her of the valve surgery she had last summer. Repeat neuropsychiatric testing with the PHD is set for next year, and she knows she will do better than she did the last time. The blockages in her neck are still at 20–49 percent, but she knows to give years of LDL around the 50–70 range before expecting any changes there. The final thing she noted was that she dreams again. The **DPC** indicated that it could be simply that now she remembers her dreams.

In a world of so many opinions and ideas, it is quite impossible that everyone would agree with me. Even as a house can be constructed on the outside to look the same as the neighbor's, the interior design, the painting, the colors, the schemes of furniture are all going to be different inside. Different individuals are unique. One person's home is much different from another's. The world would not be the same if everyone's home had to be identical. Removing the unique aspects of what we call home would simply negate our ability to have a home. You are one of a kind. There are different ways of seeing things, and this book is simply my way.

I have been working on this project for years—now I believe I need to get this information into your hands. A work in progress is never really completed. I hope you appreciate how fast information changes our interpretation of the things around us. Together we can be sure you are able to weather the storm of health care—and do the best we can to get you good medical care.

Notes

1 http://circ.ahajournals.org/cgi/content/full/121/7/e46.
2 http://www.census.gov/main/www/popclock.html.
3 U.S. National Center for Health Statistics, "Deaths: Final Data for 2007, *National Vital Statistics Reports (NVSR)* 58, no. 19, (May 2010).
4 D. Lloyd-Jones, R. Adams, M. Carnethon, et al. *Heart Disease and Stroke Statistics—2009 Update: A report from the American heart association statistics committee and stroke statistics subcommittee circulation* (2009); 199: e21-181.
5 Charlton Heston has Alzheimer's symptoms. August 9, 2002. CNN.com.
6 *Life: Gone Too Soon,* Volume 10, #11 (2010).
7 *Life: Gone Too Soon,* Volume 10, #11 (2010).
8 http://www.forbes.com/sites/investopedia/2011/10/06/how-much-would-steve-jobs-be-worth-today/.
9 *Cancer Facts & Figures 2010.* Besides lung cancer, tobacco use also causes increased risk for cancers of the mouth, lips, nasal cavity (nose) and sinuses, larynx (voice box), pharynx

(throat), esophagus (swallowing tube), stomach, pancreas, kidney, bladder, uterine cervix, and acute myeloid leukemia.

10 *Cancer Facts & Figures 2010.* In the United States, tobacco use is responsible for nearly one in five deaths; this equaled about 443,000 early deaths each year from 2000 to 2004.

11 *Cancer Facts & Figures 2010.* Tobacco use accounts for at least 30 percent of all cancer deaths and 87 percent of lung cancer deaths.

12 A. Brander, P. Viikinkoski, J. Tuuhea, L. Voutilainen, L. Kivisaari, J. Clin, "Clinical versus ultrasound examination of the thyroid gland in common clinical practice," *Ultrasound* (January 20, 1992):37–42.

13 U.S. Preventive Services Task Force (USPSTF), *Guide to Clinical Preventive Services: Report of the U.S. Preventive Services Task Force,* 2nd ed. (1996). Quote: "Screening asymptomatic adults or children for thyroid cancer using either neck palpation or ultrasonography is not recommended."

14 Waun Ki Hong, *Cancer Medicine,* eighth ed.:1.

15 http://www.utahhealthcareinitiative.com/blog/2011/06/14/primary-care-and-health-system-reform/.

16 A.J. Orehek, MD., *The Micron Stroke Hypothesis of Alzheimer's Disease and Dementia. The Journal of Medical Hypothesis.* 78.5(2012):562-70. Doi:10.1016/j.mehy.2012.01.020.

17 USPSTF 2011: 54.

18 Doi:10.1016/j.mehy.2012.01.020.

19 Quote: "The price of health care is one of the most punishing costs for families, businesses, and our government ... The insurance companies continue to ration health care ... That's the status quo in America and it's a status quo that's unsustainable"—Barack Obama. http://politcalticker.blogs.cnn.com/2010/03/08/obama-slams-health-insurance-companies.

20 "Patrick Swayze Dies of Cancer at 57," September 14, 2009, CNN.com.

21 Ian Halperin, *Brangelina: The Untold Story of Brad Pitt and Angelina Jolie* (Montreal: Transit Publishing Inc., 2009).

22 http://www.heart.org/HEARTORG/General/History-of-the-American-Heart-Association_UCM_308120.

23 Eckhart Tolle, *The Power of Now: A Guide to Spiritual Enlightenment,* 2005.

24 http://www.utahhealthcareinitiative.com/blog/2011/06/14/primary-care-and-health-system-reform.

25 "Hospitalists Should Jump on Transitions of Care Train Now to Help Solve Rehospitalization Problems," *The Hospitalist* (2011), 15(2):1–7.

26 JPA Ioannidis, "Why Most Published Research Findings Are False," *PLoS Med,* 2(8): e124, doi:10.1371/journal.pmed.0020124.

27 https://www.theabpm.org/aboutus.cfm.

28 https://www.theabpm.org/aboutus.cfm.

29 NIH, "NIH Consensus Development Conference Statement on Preventing Alzheimer's Disease and Cognitive Decline," *NIH Consensus and State-of-the-Science Statements* 27 (April 26–28, 2010).

30 2005 paper in *PLoS Medicine* by John Ioannidis. He had trouble proving his point in his study.

31 http://www.fda.gov/Drugs/DrugSafety/ucm293101.htm

32 USPTF recommendation on testicular cancer, 2011.

33 In 1999, the Institute of Medicine (IOM) issued its report, "To Err Is Human: Building a Safer Health System." The report estimated that in American hospitals, 44,000–98,000 people were dying each year due to preventable errors.

34 http://circ.ahajournals.org/cgi/content/full/121/7/e46.

35 Schousboe and Kerlikowski, "Personalizing Mammography by Breast Density and Other Risk Factors for Breast Cancer: Analysis of Health Benefits and Cost-Effectiveness," *Annals of Internal Medicine* 155, no. 1:10–20.

36 *Third Report of the Expert Panel on Detection, Evaluation, and Treatment of High Blood Cholesterol in Adults* (Adult Treatment Panel III), The Guidelines. Published in *JAMA* (2001):285:2486–2497.

37 Heart Protection Study Collaborative Group MRC/BHF, "Heart Protection Study of Cholesterol Lowering with Simvastatin

In 20,536 High-Risk Individuals: A Randomised Placebo-Controlled Trial," *The Lancet* 360, no. 9326 (2002):7–22.

38 C. P. Cannon, E. Braunwald, C. H. McCabe, D. J. Rader, J. L. Rouleau, R. Belder, S.V . Joyal, K. A. Hill, M. A. Pfeffer, and A. M. Skene, "Pravastatin or Atorvastatin Evaluation and Infection Therapy-Thrombolysis in Myocardial Infarction."

22 Investigators. Intensive versus Moderate Lipid Lowering with Statins after Acute Coronary Syndromes," *New England Journal of Medicine* (2004):350:1495–1504.

39 DOI: 10.1161/01.CIR.0000133317.49796.0E.

40 R. Schmidt et al., "MRI-Detected White Matter Lesions: Do They Really Matter?", *J Neural Transm* 118 (May 2011) 673–81. Epub 2011 Feb 22. Division of Special Neurology, Department of Neurology, Medical University of Graz, Graz, Austria. reinhold.schmidt@medunigraz.at.

41 Dr. Victoria Vetter, quoted in "Teen Athletes' Hearts in Danger," by Mary Brophy Marcus. *USA TODAY* (March 8, 2011):7D.

42 AHA/ASA, *Guidelines for Prevention of Stroke in Patients with Ischemic Stroke or Transient Ischemic Attack* (2006):37:577–617, doi: 10.1161/01.STR.0000199147.30016.74.

43 "Infectious Diseases," *The Lancet* 11, (March 2011):181–189, doi:10.1016/S1473-3099(10)70314-5. Quote: "Implementation of guidelines for management of possible multidrug-resistant pneumonia in intensive care: an observational, multicentre cohort study. Interpretation: Because adherence with empirical treatment was associated with increased mortality, we recommend a randomized trial be done before further implementation of these guidelines."

44 Ruth Purtilo, *Ethical Dimensions in the Health Professions*, 2nd ed. (Philadelphia: W.B. Saunders Company, 1992).

45 K. Paul Stoller (MD, FACH), January 13, 2009 "The history of vaccine is littered with horrible mistakes and skullduggery—from the SV40 virus given to millions in the polio vaccine to the continued use of mercury and other heavy metals. The fact is even the best MMR vaccine is contaminated with avian retro virus and reverse transcriptase. This is criminal!"

and "The truth that vaccine policy is not about science or safety but about money and politics is finally seeing the light of day." Rotarix vaccine is DNA from porcine circovirus 1 (PCV-1), on March 22, 2010—caused contamination of the vaccine.

46 Charles P. Vega, MD, *Do Healthy Adults Really Need a Flu Shot? A Best Evidence Review*, Authors and Disclosures Posted December 17, 2010.

47 Vega, *Do Healthy Adults Really Need a Flu Shot?*

48 Allen Chase , "Magic Shots: A Human and Scientific Account of the Long and Continuing Struggle to Eradicate Infectious Diseases by Vaccination."1982, p. 81. RE: shared needles.

49 Alzheimer's disease international, "global impact of dementia."

50 Z. Arvanitakis, MD, MS; J.A. Schneider, MD, MS; R. S. Wilson, PhD; J. L. Bienias, ScD; J. F. Kelly, MD; D. A. Evans, MD; D. A. Bennett, MD; "Statins, Incident Alzheimer Disease, Change in Cognitive Function, and Neuropathology," *Neurology* 70 (May 6, 2008):1801.

51 Manuel B. Graeber, *Lois Alzheimer (1864–1915)*, http://www.ibro.info/Pub_Main_Display.asp?Main_Id=34.

52 Qinghai Zhang, Evan T. Powers, Jorge Nieva, Mary E. Huff, Maria A. Dendle, Jan Bieschke, Charles G. Glabe, Albert Eschenmoser, Paul Wentworth, Jr., Richard A. Lerner, and Jeffery W. Kelly, "Metabolite-Initiated Protein Misfolding May Trigger Alzheimer's Disease," *Proceedings of the National Academy of Sciences* (March 15–19, 2004), http://dx.doi.org/10.1073/pnas.040092410.

53 American Society for Investigative Pathology, "Heme Oxygenase-1 is Associated with the Neurofibrillary Pathology of Alzheimer's Disease," *American Journal of Pathology* 145, no. 1 (July 1994).

54 Roy Yaari, MD, and Jody Corey-Bloom, MD, PhD, "Alzheimer's Disease," posted 03/07/2007, *Semin Neurol.* 27, no. 1 (Thieme Medical Publisher, 2007):32–41.

55 P. Tiraboschi, L. A. Hansen, L. J. Thal, J. Corey-Bloom, "The Importance of Neuritic Plaques and Tangles to the

Development and Evolution of AD," *Neurology* 62 (June 8, 2004)1984–9.

56 L. Kuller, "Statins and Dementia," *Current Atherosclerosis Reports* 9(2007):154–161.

57 Clifford R. Jack Jr., et al., "Introduction to the Recommendations from the National Institute on Aging and the Alzheimer's Association Workgroups on Diagnostic Guidelines for Alzheimer's Disease," *Alzheimer's and Dementia: The Journal of the Alzheimer's Association.*

58 Guy M. McKhann and David S. Knopman, et al., "The Diagnosis of Dementia Due to Alzheimer's Disease: Recommendations from the National Institute on Aging and the Alzheimer's Association Workgroup."

59 Marilyn S. Albert, et al., "The Diagnosis of Mild Cognitive Impairment Due to Alzheimer's Disease: Recommendations from the National Institute on Aging and Alzheimer's Association Workgroup."

60 Reisa A. Sperling, et al., "Toward Defining the Preclinical Stages of Alzheimer's Disease: Recommendations from the National Institute on Aging and the Alzheimer's Association Workgroup."

61 *NIH Consensus and State-of-the-Science Statements* 27 (April 26–28, 2010).

62 Thomas W. Mitchell, et al., "Novel Method to Quantify Neuropil Threads in Brains from Elders with or without Cognitive Impairment," *Journal of Histochemisty and Cytochemistry* 12 (2000):1627–1637.

63 http://www.strokecenter.org/patients/stats.htm.

64 David Salat, "Prefrontal Gray and White Matter Volumes in Health Aging and Alzheimer Disease," *Arch Neurology* 56 (Mar 1999):338–344.

65 Lewis H. Kuller, "Statins and Dementia," *Current Atherosclerosis Reports* 9, no. 2:154–161, doi: 10.1007/s11883-007-0012-9.

66 Edward M. DeSimonell (US pharmacist), "Alzheimers disease increasing numbers, but no cure," posted 2/9/2011.

67 Li, G, MD, "Statin Therapy Is Associated with Reduced Neuropathologic Changes of Alzheimer's Disease," *Neurology* (2007)69:878–885.

68 S. C. Johnston, D. R. Gress, W. S. Browner, and S. Sidney, "Short-Term Prognosis after Emergency Department Diagnosis of TIA," *JAMA 284* (2000): 2901–2906.

69 doi: 10.1161/STROKEAHA.108.19221.

70 K. L. Furie, et al., "Guidelines for the Prevention of Stroke in Patients with Stroke or Transient Ischemic Attack: A Guideline for Health-Care Professionals from the American Heart Association/American Stroke Association," *Stroke* 42 (Jan 2011):227–276. Epub 2010 Oct 21.

71 L. B. Goldstein, R. Adams, M.J. Alberts, et al. "Primary Prevention of Ischemic Stroke: A Guideline From the American Heart Association/American Stroke Association Stroke Council: Cosponsored by the Atherosclerotic Peripheral Vascular Disease Interdisciplinary Working Group; Cardiovascular Nursing Council; Clinical Cardiology Council; Nutrition, Physical Activity, and Metabolism Council; and the Quality of Care and Outcomes Research Interdisciplinary Working Group," *Stroke* 37 (2006). Published online May 4, 2006, ahead of print. Accessed August 14, 2006. Available at: http://stroke.ahajournals.org/.

72 L. B. Goldstein, R. Adams, K. Becker, et al., "Primary Prevention of Ischemic Stroke: A Statement for Healthcare Professionals from the Stroke Council of the American Heart Association," *Stroke* 32 (2001):280–299.

73 R. L. Sacco, AHA, et al., "Guidelines for Prevention of Stroke in Patients with Ischemic Stroke or Transient Ischemic Attack: A Statement for Healthcare Professionals from the American Heart Association/American Stroke Association Council on Stroke," *Stroke* 37 (2006):577–617.

74 doi: 10.1161/STROKEAHA.107.189063.

75 Page 73 of the 2011 guide.

76 http://www.nia.nih.gov/Alzheimers/AlzheimersInformation/Diagnosis.

77 Yulin ge, et al., "Age-Related Total Gray Matter and White Matter Changes in Normal Adult Brain. Part 1: Volumetric MR Imaging Analysis," *Ajnr Am J Neuroradiology* 23:1327–1333. (2002).

78 J. C. Moms, MD; A. Heyman, MD; R. C. Mohs, PhD; J. P. Hughes, MS; G. van Belle, PhD; G. Fillenbaum, PhD; E. D. Mellits, ScD; and C. Clark, MD; *The Consortium to Establish a Registry for Alzheimer's Disease (CERAD), Part I: Clinical and Neuropsychological Assessment of Alzheimer's Disease.*

79 S. S. Mirra, MD, et al., "The Consortium to Establish a Registry for Alzheimer's Disease (CERAD) Part II: Standardization of the Neuropathologic Assessment of Alzheimer's Disease," *Neurology* 41 (April 1991):479–486.

80 http://www.nia.nih.gov/Alzheimers/Publications/stages. htm.

81 http://www.nia.nih.gov/Alzheimers/Publications/stages. htm.

82 http://www.nia.nih.gov/Alzheimers/Publications/stages. htm.

83 A&E Television Networks, *Hoarders*, 2011, http://www.aetv. com/hoarders.

84 John J.P. Kastelein, MD, PhD, Fatima Akdim, MD, Erik S. G. Stroes, MD, PhD, Aeilko H. Zwinderman, PhD, Michiel L. Bots, MD, PhD, Anton F.H. Stalenhoef, MD, PhD, F.R.C.P., Frank L.J. Visseren, MD, PhD, Eric J.G. Sijbrands, MD, PhD, Mieke D. Trip, MD, PhD, Evan A. Stein, MD, PhD, Daniel Gaudet, MD, PhD, Raphael Duivenvoorden, MD, Enrico P. Veltri, MD, A. David Marais, MD, PhD, and Eric de Groot, MD, PhD for the ENHANCE Investigators, "Simvastatin with or without Ezetimibe in Familial Hypercholesterolemia," *New England Journal of Medicine* 358 (April 3, 2008)1431–1443.

85 D. A. Fishman, L. Cohen, S.V. Blank, et al., "The Role of Ultrasound Evaluation in the Detection of Early-Stage Epithelial Ovarian Cancer," *Am J Obstet Gynecol* 192, no. 4, (2005):1214–1221 (discussion 21–22).

86 I.J. Jacobs and U. Menon, "Progress and Challenges in Screening for Early Detection of Ovarian Cancer," *Mol Cell Proteomics* 3, no. 4 (2004):355–366.

87 B. A. Goff, L. S. Mandel, C.H. Melancon, et al., "Frequency of Symptoms of Ovarian Cancer in Women Presenting to Primary Care Clinics," *JAMA 291, no.22* (2004):2705–2712.

88 http://tcrc.acor.org/l6.html.

89 http://www.goal-setting-college.com/inspiration/lance-armstrong.

90 http://www.seer.cancer.gov/csr/1975_2005/results_merged/sect_25_testis.pdf.

91 Screening for testicular cancer part of USPSTF 2011.

92 http://www.uspreventiveservicestaskforce.org/3rduspstf/testicular/testiculup.htm.

93 http://tcrc.acor.org/lance.html.

94 Todd Neale, "AHA: Vital Elements Often Missing from Sports Physicals," *MedPage Today* (November 15, 2011).

95 S. Ebrahim, F. Taylor, K. Ward, A. Beswick, M. Burke, and G. Davey Smith, "Multiple risk factor interventions for primary prevention of coronary heart disease," *Cochrane Database of Systematic Reviews* 1 (2011):Art. No.: CD001561, doi: 10.1002/14651858.CD001561.pub3.

96 MP Heron, DL Hoyert, SL Murphy, JQ Xu, KD Kochanek, B Tejada-Vera. "Deaths: Final Data for 2006," *National Vital Statistics Reports* 57, no.14 (2009).

97 John Fauber, "Doctor Fired after Revealing Testing Flaws," *Milwaukee Sentinel Journal/MedPage Today* (January 15, 2011).

98 John J. P. Kastelein, MD, et al., "Simvastatin with or without Ezetimibe in Familial Hypercholesterolemia," 1431–1443.

99 MUST PULL A study, I don't care if it is a rat study that shows how there is 'endoreplication' of arterial blood smooth vessel cells. They are to replicate their DNA without cell division. "smooth muscle cells may endoreplicate, that is their DNA is replicated without cell division" as it is related to HTN.

100 V. Roger, A. Go, D. Lloyd-Jones, et al., "Heart Disease and Stroke statistics—2011 Update: A Report from the American

Heart Association Statistics Committee and Stroke Statistics Subcommittee," *Circulation* 123 (2011)e1–e192.

101 http://www.cdc.gov/bloodpressure/facts.htm.

102 World Health Organization, International Society of Hypertension writing group, "2003 Statement on Management of Hypertension," *Journal of Hypertension* 21 (2003):1983-1992.

103 http://www.cdc.gov/bloodpressure/facts.htm.

104 The ACCORD Study Group, "Effect of Intensive Blood Pressure Control in Type 2 Diabetes Mellitus," *New England Journal of Medicine* 363 (April 29, 2010): 17.

105 http://www.healthimaging.com/index.php?option=com_ articles&view=article&id=22380:ny-cards-scramble-to-re-view-4000-unread-echos-at-harlem-hospital.

106 L. B. Woolner, M. L. Lemmon, O. H. Beahrs, et al., "Occult Papillary Carcinoma of the Thyroid Gland: A Study of 140 Cases Observed in a 30-Year Period," *J Clin Endocr Metab* 20 (1960):89–105.

107 2010 cancer facts and figures (same as the other reference).

108 Bookshelf ID: NBK15464.

109 "AACE/AAES Medical/surgical guidelines for clinical prac-tice: management of thyroid carcinoma," *Endocrine Practice* 7, (May/June 2001).

110 American Association of Clinical Endocrinologists, as-sociation MEDICI endocrinology, and European Thyroid Association medical guidelines for clinical practice for the diagnosis and management of thyroid nodule *Endocrine Practice* 12 (Jan-Feb, 2006):63–102.

111 Benny Evangelista, "Apple's Jobs Has Cancerous Tumor Removed," *San Francisco Chronicle*, (August 2, 2004):A1. http://www.sfgate.com/cgi-bin/article.cgi?file=/ c/a/2004/08/02/MNGMJ816F41.DTL.

112 Page 36 of USPSTF 2011.

113 Naheed R. Abbasi Molly Yancovitz, Dina Gutkowicz-Krusin, Katherine S. Panageas, Martin C. Mihm, Paul Googe, Roy King, Victor Prieto, Iman Osman, Robert J. Friedman, Darrell S. Rigel, Alfred W. Kopf, and David Polsky, "Utility of Lesion

Diameter in the Clinical Diagnosis of Cutaneous Melanoma," *Archives of Dermatology* 144 (April, 2008):469–74.

114 D.S. Rigel, "Epidemiology of Melanoma," *Seminars in Cutaneous Medicine & Surgery* 29 (2010): 204 (#J0206228).

115 http://www.ahrq.gov/uspstf home page (Accessed on 10-22-11).

116 http://www.ahrq.gov/clinic/pocketgd1011/pocket-gd1011.pdf (accessed on 2-13-11).

117 L.B. Squiers, D.J. Holden, S.E. Dolina, A.E. Kim, C.M. Bann, and J.M. Renaud, "The public's response to the U.S. Preventive Services Task Force's 2009 recommendations on mammography screening," *American Journal of Preventive Medicine* 40 (May, 2011): 497–504.

118 Perry Potter and Patricia Potter, *Fundamentals of Nursing* (2009).

119 *Annals of Internal Medicine* 149, (November 4, 2008): 635.

120 Colorectal Cancer: Risk Factors and Recommendations for Early Detection, THOMAS E. READ, M.D., and IRA J. KODNER, M.D., Washington University School of Medicine, St. Louis, Missouri, Am Fam physician. 1999 Jun 1; 59(11):3083-3092.

121 USPSTF summary of breast cancer screening evaluation.

122 http://www.ncbi.nlm.nih.gov/books/NBK36398/#ch3.s7.

123 "Canadian National Breast Screening Study-2: 13-year results of a randomized trial in women aged 50-59 years" *J Natl Cancer Inst.* 92 (Sept., 2000): 1490–9.

124 Clinical breast examination section of 2011 USPSTF recommendations.

125 Digital mammography section of 2011 USPSTF recommendations.

126 MRI part of USPSTF 2011 recommendations.

127 *Rudolph the Red-Nosed Reindeer* by Rankin/Bass. First aired December 6, 1964 on NBC.

128 M.A. Creager, J.L. Halperin, and A.D. Whittemore, "Aneurysmal disease of the aorta and its branches," *Vascular Medicine* (New York: Little, Brown, 1996).

129 COPD Will Cost U.S. Over $800 Billion Over Next 20 Years Main Category: COPD Also Included In: Public Health Article

Date: 30 May 2006 - 0:00 PDT http://www.medicalnewstoday.com/releases/44235.php (accessed 6-15-2011).

130 Page 36 of the USPSTF 2011.

131 http://www.ahrq.gov/clinic/pocketgd1011/pocketgd1011.pdf.

132 American Cancer Society. Cancer Facts & Figures 2010. Atlanta: American Cancer Society; 2010.

133 USPSTF page ovarian cancer 2011.

134 http://www.cdc.gov/nchs/data/nvsr/nvsr60/nvsr60_04.pdf.

135 K. M. Woo, J. I. Schneider, "High-Risk Chief Complaints I: Chest Pain—The Big Three." *Emerg. Med. Clin. North Am.* 27 (November 2009): 685–712.

136 https://www.cms.gov/ReportsTrustFunds/downloads/tr2011.pdf (accessed 7-20-11). 2011 Annual Report of the Boards of Trustees of the Federal Hospital Insurance and Federal Supplementary Medical Insurance Trust Funds.